The Conception I

Dr Larisa Corda is an obstetrician and gynaecologist, with a specialist interest in fertility. She qualified as a medical doctor from Imperial College, London, and has trained and practised in the UK and Australia. She believes in a mind–body holistic approach to well-being and fertility, which addresses the physical, mental and spiritual dimensions of health. Her research interests include the effect of stress on reproductive outcomes and older-age motherhood. She also has a focus on improving the global injustice of inequity through facilitating access to reproductive care.

Larisa is a passionate women's rights ambassador, and she has played roles on a number of charities, such as UN Women, the Circle, Saying Goodbye, Kicks Count and Endometriosis UK. She received the WeAre TheCity Rising Star in healthcare award in 2020, and in 2022 she was nominated for a BBC Radio London Make a Difference key worker award, for her work on the frontline during the pandemic. She regularly appears and advises as a women's health, fertility and pregnancy expert in the media, including TV and radio. Her uniquely devised programme for conception and pregnancy, The Conception Plan, was aired on *This Morning*. She is dedicated to dismantling stigmas and taboos so often found within female health, and to empowering women and men over their fertility and wellness.

The Conception Plan

The Science-backed Guide to Fertility and Becoming a Parent

DR LARISA CORDA

PENGUIN LIFE

AN IMPRINT OF

PENGUIN BOOKS

PENGUIN LIFE

UK | USA | Canada | Ireland | Australia
India | New Zealand | South Africa

Penguin Life is part of the Penguin Random House group of companies
whose addresses can be found at global.penguinrandomhouse.com.

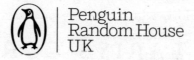

First published 2023

001

Set in 12/15pt Dante MT Pro
Typeset by Jouve (UK), Milton Keynes
Printed and bound in Great Britain by Clays Ltd, Elcograf S.p.A.

The authorized representative in the EEA is Penguin Random House Ireland,
Morrison Chambers, 32 Nassau Street, Dublin D02 YH68

A CIP catalogue record for this book is available from the British Library

ISBN: 978–0–241–52446–6

www.greenpenguin.co.uk

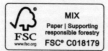

Penguin Random House is committed to a
sustainable future for our business, our readers
and our planet. This book is made from Forest
Stewardship Council® certified paper.

To my Great-Aunt Masa, who left this Earthly realm during the writing of this book, but who will forever remain one of my greatest teachers. Her greatness came not just from her age and experience, but by virtue of her wisdom and love, which had an immeasurable impact on my life and, for someone as humble as she was, I can see her on the other side telling me off for making a fuss over her. Yet this book wouldn't be here, were it not for some of the most important things I learned from her: that in our brokenness lie our very gifts; that love transcends all boundaries; that family is everything; and that our souls are capable of miracles we can't even imagine until they happen. She had the heart of a rebel, which recognized a kindred spirit in me, though she rarely let me know it. This 'book written in the woods' is a tribute to her and to her enduring legacy as a mother, grandmother, sister, daughter and great-aunt.

Contents

Contents

Foreword

The conception of this book was a committed labour of love, which would not have been possible without the support and help of various individuals who guided me in birthing it into the world. The idea behind it was planted in 2019, when The Conception Plan was a series of ideas that arose from my practice and experience over the years, helping to guide three couples who applied to be coached by me on the TV show *This Morning*.

As I sit here in the heart of Dorset, writing the concluding part of my book, I can't help reflecting on what feels like a full 360-degree moment. When I first shared The Conception Plan in its embryonic stages, it was with the aim of bringing hope to as many people as possible who were struggling to conceive, by helping those who had agreed to have their journey to parenthood broadcast on TV and so reaching all those who would not have access to this information. This is when I first met Kathryn and Dan, whom I brought to this very same sanctuary nestled in the small town of Sherborne, near the magical Cerne Abbas Giant, to integrate this new approach. Only a few weeks afterwards, they found themselves pregnant with their first child, Freddie. I had no idea back then that this would go on to inspire a book, and would also enable many of you who wrote to me afterwards to have your own miracles unfold, too.

Often the stories you shared – and continue to share – had a common thread of many years of pain and disempowerment, being left feeling helpless and lost in a process that felt beyond your control, with all the answers seemingly to be found outside you. I hope that whether it's through reading this book or watching the TV segment, or both, you've been able to see quite how much there is that you can do, how many of the answers lie within you and how they're directly accessible, if you're willing to view your health and fertility through the lens of holism. Most of all, I hope you get to realize the difference that you can make.

My big passion is to empower people to be the healthiest and most fertile expressions of themselves, from the inside out, and to help build families where children are a natural expression of this awareness. This is why I created The Conception Plan, an integrated, scientifically spiritual approach to conceiving, where I share all my learnings and teach you to give birth first to the parent you want to be, before I help you to have a child. My experience of working with various patients over the years has shown me that infertility almost always reveals a space, and a place where healing needs to occur on an emotionally ingrained level. It often involves dealing with issues related to our inner child: the times when we didn't feel safe, experienced trauma and didn't deal with it, or the emotional wounds that we accumulated as a result of not having our needs met. The process of conception requires that we tend to our inner child first and transfigure our life experiences and the etchings they left on our bodies and nervous systems, so that we can become parents from a place of wholeness. This is precisely why an integrated approach that places as much emphasis on the mind and emotions as it does on the body is vital when it comes to treating infertility.

The paradigm that modern medicine seems to be built upon – which is that of providing a fix to a problem – doesn't hold space for the idea that humans are capable of their own transformation and healing. And so when it comes to conditions such as infertility, although we may have technologies such as IVF that can help, there is very little out there recognizing that people are often capable of healing their infertility from within, and that the condition can offer an important window into the biopsychosocial state of a person, with opportunities to heal and transform. The new age of medicine is about empowering people to understand that disease is a manifestation of our environment interacting with our genes, and is controlled by how we live. This means that we often have the power to do something about it when we recognize symptoms and conditions as expressions of the complex biological landscape within our bodies, shaped by our emotions and our past experiences.

This book was written on sacred spiritual land in Somerset, on a sheep farm, where I observed the incredible power of the natural world birthing new life – and I'm sure it's no coincidence that my book took nine months to gestate into an initial manuscript. During this time I became aware of the need to change the narrative around infertility and start a different model of healthcare focused on preconception, to help people have a more empowered approach to conceiving, combining my passion for both science and spirit. The bridge between these two worlds has always seemed so natural to me, and yet it's incredible to consider how separate and polarized these two modalities have become in our modern world. How often has spirituality been dismissed as woo-woo and charlatan, and science been seen as arrogant and patriarchal, by those in seemingly opposite camps?

The truth is that both carry generations of wisdom, and both are an integral part of our humanness. If we view our bodies as nothing more than science, we completely disconnect from the multidimensional nature of who we are and the multifaceted world we exist in. And so, as we see with a lot of mainstream medicine where our emotions still aren't accepted as part of our health, and where we continue to treat our minds and bodies as separate autonomous entities, we seem to be falling short of being able to necessarily cure people.

PART 1
The Fundamentals

Prologue: where it all began

One sunny Sunday morning a message appeared on my phone. It was a photograph of a positive pregnancy test, two unmistakable dark lines. Two lines whose deceptive simplicity concealed three preceding years of disappointment and heartache.

The pregnancy test belonged to Kathryn and Dan, a couple I coached on the TV show *This Morning*. Only weeks earlier, desperate to conceive, they had contacted the programme to apply to be a part of The Conception Plan (TCP), which I had created to help all those struggling to conceive and who, in many cases, had been prevented from seeking help on the NHS. Following a carefully tailored overhaul of their lifestyle and some coaching, here they were, on the cusp of a new chapter, expecting their first baby. This was their first-ever positive pregnancy test, and I was the first person they were sharing their incredible news with.

It was real: Kathryn was pregnant. That same year, just in time for Christmas, she and Dan brought into the studio their miracle baby, Freddie, who had been born earlier in December. He lay cradled in his parents' arms, owning his moment in the spotlight, blissfully unaware of what it took to bring him into the world.

Kathryn and Dan's story had started three years before they met me. One in seven couples struggles to conceive. If that's you, you'll know how that struggle can be painfully long and is almost always all-consuming. Before trying to get pregnant, Kathryn had been on the contraceptive pill for a long time. She assumed, like a lot of women I speak to, that after stopping it, she would get pregnant soon afterwards.

Instead Kathryn found that her periods were irregular. Eventually she was diagnosed with polycystic ovaries, a condition that affects up to 25 per cent of women. It can mean that a woman doesn't ovulate and so finds it more difficult to become pregnant. On top of that, Dan was diagnosed with a low sperm count, as well as a groin hernia and a varicocele (enlarged veins in the scrotum), all of which can affect the quality of sperm.

With a body mass index (BMI) of more than forty, Kathryn was – sadly and unfairly – excluded from being able to access fertility treatment on the NHS, including basic advice about what to do. So she and Dan continued to struggle without help, until she applied to *This Morning* to seek assistance from me.

I started Kathryn and Dan on The Conception Plan. As you'll discover, it has five pillars – nutrition, exercise, stress management, toxin-free living, and sex and relationships – and holistically combines cutting-edge Western science with ancient Eastern wisdom. Together we made drastic changes to the couple's eating habits, starting them on a predominantly plant-based diet with plenty of organic, seasonal, wholesome foods. They started drinking filtered water. Their exercise included a mixture of cardiovascular and resistance training, with the aim of reaching 150 minutes per week. We replaced home cleaning equipment, detergents, soaps and shampoos with those that mini-mized any hormone-disrupting chemicals.

Finally we looked at the issue of chronic stress: how it was showing up in their lives and how they were managing it. Under my guidance, Kathryn and Dan left the bustle of life in Bournemouth to visit a holistic retreat in the depths of Dorset, where they experienced treatments – ranging from reiki and crystal healing to shamanism – to help them explore a whole new dimension in terms of shifting their stress and accessing their mind and emotions to help them heal.

It was then that I had my goosebumps moment, sensing they were on the threshold of becoming parents and feeling, as well as witness-ing, a physical, emotional and spiritual shift occur in the couple. That weekend, when I spoke to Kathryn, suddenly all the years of built-up emotions that she'd been carrying gave way to tears, as she visibly released the energetic blocks that had stopped her from manifest-ing the thing she most desired in the world. She and Dan not only readied their bodies and their environment to conceive a baby, but also uncluttered their emotional space, thereby expanding their cap-acity to receive. My intuition told me that they were on the brink of a life-changing moment, co-creating their future and opening themselves up to new possibilities. And it was a few short weeks later that the couple discovered they were expecting.

How did they do this, without assisted reproductive treatment? They applied the five pillars of The Conception Plan to heal on a physical, mental *and* emotional level. They used each one of the pillars to reset and optimize their general health and fertility and to create a new state of well-being, embodying what it meant to be fertile in all aspects of their lives.

This book is here to help you achieve the same sort of healing and change. I believe that, with enough care and dedication, it's possible to rewrite your reproductive destiny. Kathryn and Dan had a lot working against them, including multiple medical issues. Not many people would have betted on them having a biological child naturally. Yet this is exactly what happened. With the help of The Conception Plan, they went on to reprogramme their destiny, and ultimately their long-term health and wellness.

Introduction: what to expect from The Conception Plan

Welcome to The Conception Plan. Whether you're currently trying to get pregnant, are going through IVF (*in vitro* fertilization) or are interested in making sure you'll be ready to carry a baby at some point in the future, this book is for you.

Over the years I've helped build many families and have assisted them in birthing their babies. I bring to this book not only my clinical and scientific experience, but also my spiritual understanding and training in what it means to be truly whole, healthy and fertile. I'll give you some clear medical and lifestyle advice for wherever you are in your journey, but I will also help you see some aspects of yourself that you might not know are important to your health and fertility. In fact a lot of mainstream medicine hasn't yet understood how important these aspects are. The changes that you'll make will be simple, implementable and often inexpensive. But, over time, they will have a big impact.

This book bridges the gap between science and spirit. It's a *scientifically spiritual* guide for conception – my unique and proven approach to becoming pregnant. It will show you how to access the best of both worlds when it comes to conceiving, and how conception is a process that occurs as a result of the path of conscious evolution leading to parenthood. This is what I refer to as 'conscious conception'.

Conventional medicine doesn't do much to teach us how eggs and sperm can be *optimized*, how to improve the conditions for natural conception and how so much of the power to conceive lies within our own sphere of influence. These ideas may sound a little different from what you're used to hearing, but in The Conception Plan you'll discover that they are firmly rooted in science. As you will come to see, many concepts that were previously thought of as only spiritual are now part of a New Age of science.

This book will also show you how my approach deconstructs health into its many contributory factors. This will help you manage any condition or issue that may be underpinning your own or your partner's ability to conceive. It will also build foundations to navigate your health for the rest of your life, including during the post-natal period, any subsequent pregnancies and even the menopause.

Why do we need The Conception Plan?

One in seven couples has trouble conceiving, and this number is growing, according to a 2019 report from the US Centers for Disease Control and Prevention. Not all of this is down to ageing parents (and, as we'll explore, in many cases you can actually have control over some of the effects of ageing).

Now that we have IVF, many clinics don't offer investigations into the subtler causes of infertility. Why would they, when there's a method that can potentially resolve the issue and save time for the patient? The simple reason why I don't agree with this approach is that having a baby doesn't necessarily make you fertile. But committing to a process where you effectively birth a healthier version of yourself prior to becoming a parent, expanding the possibilities available to you and addressing all aspects of your physical, emotional and spiritual wellness, will lead to being fertile in all areas of your life, in addition to helping you birth a baby into the world.

Up to one-third of people have what the medical profession continues to call 'unexplained infertility'. This means there seems to be no obvious clinical cause, despite the usual fertility investigations. Very often these people are treated with assisted reproductive technologies, without finding out *why* they can't get pregnant.

However, I believe it's better to treat the root causes, rather than bypass them. All the patients I've ever met who have been diagnosed with 'unexplained infertility' want to know *what's behind it*. When you know the cause, you are far more empowered to be able to do something about it. Anyone who's been trying for a long time wants to know what they can do to make a baby happen. Everyone wants to be their most fertile and healthy and to maximize their baby's health too, whether they plan to conceive now or are thinking about a baby in the future.

Your body (unless you use a surrogate, in which case they need this book too!) will be the incubator for your future baby. What you do now will either reduce or increase the chance of successful fertilization and implantation, as well as the health of your future child. It will affect how healthy your pregnancy is and how well you feel throughout it.

Doing TCP may mean you don't need to use assisted fertility techniques such as IVF, which can be arduous as well as traumatic, and should not be used in place of treating reversible causes of infertility. And if you do still need to use assisted reproductive technology (ART), you'll improve your chances of success by investing in your health, first and foremost, which will also help reduce the number of times you may need this intervention. What you do to set the foundations before you become pregnant will pay dividends later, because the health of your baby is determined several months before you even consider conceiving. This is what ultimately co-creates your epigenetic profile (more on this later). This time of preparation is far from passive, but is rather a crucial opportunity to restructure and reshape your health as well as your life.

The way I approach fertility is quite different from what you may have been led to expect from a doctor. As well as taking into account your medical history, I'm also interested in your psychological hygiene, your thought patterns, your life experiences all the way back to your childhood, your capacity for self-love and compassion and your family relationships, as well as the most important relationship of all: the one you have with yourself. You may experience sensitivities to some of the things that you read, especially if they resonate with experiences you may have had, but that isn't a bad thing. In fact quite the opposite: it can be a really useful indicator of the places where healing needs to occur.

Research now shows that many of the reasons people aren't getting pregnant – and a lot of the ways they can improve their chances of getting pregnant – lie in their environment and habits: namely, eating, exercise, stress and exposure to many chemicals. Fertility is a balance of neurochemical, hormonal, immunological and other biological processes, all of which have important roles. As you'll find out, these can impact on egg and sperm quality, influence your genes and affect cell repair and ageing, as well as lead to localized and whole-body inflammation, metabolic dysfunction, poorer mito-chondrial function and repair, sensitization to the effect of stress on your body and impairment of the health of your microbiome (the colonies of health-promoting organisms found in the body) . . . all of which feed into your fertility and general wellness. But there are also other unseen and silent factors that affect the ability to conceive, and these relate to our minds and are not necessarily measurable, but can nonetheless leave significant imprints on the cells and tissues where fertility-related processes take place.

The Conception Plan addresses major areas where almost all of us need to improve. It isn't a case of radically overhauling everything. It's about understanding that you have the power to control so much of your own health through slow and steady adjustments in your direct environment, which will change your behaviour. This in turn will affect your long-term habits and your relationship with your mind and body.

Small steps taken each day, when they are sustained, will not only improve your fertility, but also your general sense of well-being, leaving you with more energy, better mental clarity and a fitter body and mind. I have seen this approach help and support many people in their quest to have a baby and lead a healthier life. But even beyond that, when people become truly aligned physically, mentally and spiritually, they become potent creators and manifesters of their future and their destiny.

Becoming a parent

One dictionary definition of 'fertile' is *capable of becoming a new individual*. During the preparation for becoming a parent, not only are you getting ready to make a new individual, but you're also changing and reshaping yourself.

For some people, getting pregnant can appear magically simple. For others, this is not the case: hours spent monitoring ovulation, timing sex, going from scan to scan, injecting needles into themselves and waiting for test results. It can be both emotionally and physically over-whelming. You may feel powerless, losing confidence and even identity, and damaging your self-worth and your mental health in the process.

There is no denying the fact that trying to conceive may test you in the most challenging of ways. Even the 'easiest' of fertility journeys brings with it anxieties and difficulties. And struggling to have a baby can put you in touch with your deepest vulnerabilities. The loss of control can make everything in life feel precarious and overwhelming. Any plan becomes provisional. Living in a state of anxiety, disorienta-tion and constant change becomes the new normal.

If all this sounds familiar, then I promise you it's possible to come home to yourself again. This book is about the small, steady steps you can do, on repeat, to help move you in a new direction as you regain a sense of control. Having faith in being able to adapt, make changes and get through what seem like insurmountable obstacles will help to guide you past your grief, confusion, anger and lost convictions. All you have to do, at the beginning, is commit to taking the small steps in this book. This is an act of faith. Soon you'll begin to get a glimmer of hope – and that can be all you need to keep going. This is why I created The Conception Plan, to provide something tangible in a situ-ation that can sometimes feel anything but. TCP will give you a sense of direction and purpose, enabling you to become the fittest and most thriving version of yourself. As they say, if you want to see a change in your life, you must do something different. By picking up this book, you've already shown yourself willing to commit to change.

Why are emotions important to fertility?

Whether it's treating patients with infertility or managing a woman's labour, I often learn a lot more about the patient from observation rather than from what they say. When I ask about feelings, relation-ships, previous experiences and emotions, this almost inevitably opens people up to reveal hidden fears, grief and pain, which can often be subconscious. It has become increasingly obvious to me that there are always multiple factors influencing how a woman or a man feels going into pregnancy and birth, and these can interfere with their ability to conceive, yet all too often they are completely missed by those of us in the medical profession.

But bigger than that, suppressed emotions are not innocuous. They influence a whole cascade of biological processes that create your chemical and hormonal environment, which ultimately impacts on your overall well-being and even your fertility, via epigenetics (more on this in the next chapter).

Your brain is one of the most important reproductive organs, because it directly interacts with all the other organs and oversees their behaviour. As you'll see in Chapter 2, evidence is building about the impact of the mind and previous emotional experiences on many diseases, including endometriosis and chronic pelvic pain. Mental and emotional health matters, and fertility is a place where they matter significantly.

As a doctor, I've learned that when there is a greater appreciation of the emotional context of someone's symptoms and presentation, this can lead to insights and breakthroughs in helping that person. Every case study in this book shares the emotional factors that affected the person's overall state of health and fertility. As you make your way through the book, I will encourage you to take time to consider how your own previous experiences may have shaped your emotions and your health too.

These invisible layers of old emotions and trauma may seem a million miles away from getting pregnant. But as Deepak Chopra states, we are not inside our minds, but our mind is inside us and in every single cell of our being. As I'll show you in Chapter 2, every single cell of our bodies – no matter what organ it relates to – can memorize experiences.

The miracle of life

Ancient traditions have long upheld a spiritual view of reproduction, whereas modern medicine identifies problems and provides a more mechanical solution. As useful as assisted conception methods such as IVF are, they have created a medical system where the sacred act of conceiving is treated as solely a physical process.

But conception is the unification of the body, mind and soul of two beings. It starts with the consciousness brought to the act of conceiving, leading to the fertilization of the sperm and egg, which then gives rise to a human being. It shouldn't come as a surprise that an approach involving the unification of science and spirituality is what's needed to cultivate a new understanding and awareness around conception.

Increasingly holistic methods, such as acupuncture, reiki and reflexology, are being used to help those wanting to conceive, as an add-on to medical care. The two worlds are beginning to work together, to help support the path to parenthood, but in general health too. In part it's because people are taking their health into their own hands, with greater access to a wealth of information than ever before and an interest in what complementary approaches can bring.

It's also partly because, as you'll see in Chapter 2, there are a growing number of scientific explanations for why holistic methods work. Take, for example, meditation. We now know that it has real and measurable physiological and biochemical effects in the body that can ultimately affect fertility.

WHY PRECONCEPTION STARTS AT PUBERTY

Our fertility reflects our general health and well-being, and also our emotional, mental and spiritual balance. If you were fortunate enough to receive any sort of sex education at school, the chances are that you were told how *not* to get pregnant. You were probably not made aware that conception is a finely orchestrated domino effect of fragile and precarious bodily processes.

This is why I'm passionate about speaking about fertility as early as speaking about sex. Preconception care – which really includes all the care that we invest in ourselves from the point when we become fertile – will determine not only our ability to become pregnant, but how healthy that pregnancy is, our post-natal recovery and, eventually, the symptoms that affect us during the menopause. It will also have an impact on our wider health and, as detailed in Chapter 5, any adverse events that we're exposed to at this time, and the emotional consequences they leave behind, that can set the stage for long-term disease, including infertility. As you'll see in Chapter 1, our own health impacts on the health of our children and, as science is showing, several generations of children thereafter. So you can see why I'm so passionate about getting the message out about preconception care. With enough awareness and commitment, we have the means to pass on a legacy of health to our children, no matter what may have affected us in life.

Every method, idea, intervention, process and piece of advice that I have put into TCP I use in my own life and wholeheartedly recommend to my patients. This is a fertility *lifestyle*. Each small step you take during the twelve weeks of the pillars of TCP will be building strong foundations for a happy, healthy pregnancy. As the practical, simple changes accumulate over time, you will not only notice a difference, but will also *feel different*. And as has been the case for all those I have looked after with this plan, it's not simply their health that has changed, but their whole life. When you learn the tools for co-creating a new level of health and fertility, this has the added benefit of allowing you to create circumstances in your life that are more fully aligned and true to the new version of yourself. All that's required is for you to commit to it.

The Conception Plan

Part 1 takes you through the fundamentals of my new approach to fertility, where you become empowered enough to realize that you already have all the answers you've been seeking within you and can do something about it. This is likely going to be different from a lot of the advice you've heard before. And it will probably completely change your perspective on what it takes to get pregnant. It explains the science of why fertility isn't just about a collection of eggs or the production of sperm, but about all of you as a human being: body, mind, emotions and spirit. It also explains how and why all the practical advice in Part 2 and in the 12-week plan is going to make a difference. I've found that once people are empowered with this knowledge, they are prepared to make the changes necessary, but also have the mindset and the spiritual fortitude to see it through.

Part 2 of the book explains what you can actually *do*. It starts with the key pillars: nutrition, exercise, stress management, minimizing toxin exposure, plus sex and relationships. Each section gives you scientifically proven and practical ways to get your body and mind into the best condition for conception and beyond. Putting into action the information in each of the pillars can feel overwhelming at first. That is where the next section, the 12-week plan, comes in: it breaks down all the advice into an easy-to-achieve programme. I chose twelve weeks because it's three menstrual cycles. That's how long it takes for the egg and sperm to change from being cells in storage to being ready to use. It's also the right amount of time to commit to TCP lifestyle changes and make them a way of life from then on. Three months may seem a long time, but after a few weeks, once you start to notice changes, you'll want to keep going. You'll learn various methods to tune into the subtle clues your body is giving you, such as journaling and cycle monitoring. And you'll learn how to change your mindset and your physical well-being with powerful tools, including visualization, meditation and breathwork. You'll also commit to making nutrition and exercise changes that suit you. You'll notice that I'm not overly strict, but I do give you some guidelines and options: it will become clear to you what works for *you*.

Part 3 is where the plan gets personalized. It explains and deconstructs all the physical causes that can get in the way of having a healthy baby, from polycystic ovary syndrome (PCOS) and endometriosis, to miscarriage and male factors behind infertility.

Becoming a parent is the biggest commitment you will make in your life. It makes sense that you invest as much time in preparing for this (if not more) as you would in finding the perfect job or life partner. This book is a guide to being prepared and in the best state of health possible, so that you feel confident in the approach to your pregnancy.

Your body is incredible. And you can enhance your chances of getting pregnant through thoughtful and consistent changes to your lifestyle, as well as gentle probing into how you came to be the person you are today, and into the person you want to become.

Let's get started. Start making better decisions. Start taking more powerful and courageous action. You can change your life and your health and fertility.

Infertility throws down a gauntlet for transformation, and the extent of your transformation depends on how deeply you embody the consciousness behind conception. When you do this work before bringing children into the world, you enable them to inherit a different path of evolution. The road to becoming a parent can often feel like a labyrinth: a path you trust to unfold, but with no clear vision of where it may lead. There's an entrance leading to a destination, with both tension and dynamics within it. This ancient symbol is related to the concept of wholeness, where all the meandering takes you along a purpose-driven path. The sort of path that you walk is laden with choices, and the choices you make will determine the final destination. But before you can do this journey, you first have to travel inwards, where what you learn allows you to embody wisdom and compassion for yourself. This journey is never linear, but is often rocky and turbulent as you explore your own deep-rooted emotions and their origins, taking you forward, but not before you travel inwards first.

CHAPTER 1

Epigenetics: the science behind lifestyle changes

You doubtless know that being healthy is the key to becoming, and staying, pregnant. You may know it's a good idea to eat well and exercise for the health of your future baby too. But do you know *how* what you do can transform your fertility and the baby's future health?

There's a paradigm shift happening in the way we understand genes and their impact on our health and fertility. Previously it was thought that health and fertility were determined by your genes – which you couldn't change. Now we know this isn't the case.

Epigenetics is the science of how our outer and inner environments alter the way our genes are read. And how the combination of experiences that we have and choices that we make in life effectively form our epigenome. You could describe our genes – which we inherit from our mother and father – as the recipe of who we will become; and then epigenetics is the cook who helps our body to read and create that genetic recipe.

This is a relatively new and very fast-growing area of research. For example, scientists previously thought that only 2 per cent of the human genome had a function, and 98 per cent was merely 'junk DNA'. It turns out that it's far from being junk; the majority of it has a role in gene expression – that is, how genes behave.

Epigenetics has not only formed the person we are now, but can change our future physical selves, including our future health. And (this is the mind-blowing part) epigenetic changes can also transform the genetic material we're making – our eggs or sperm – and, eventually, the future health of the baby we create. Not only can we shape and mould our own health destiny, but we can also even do the same for our children.

Epigenetics explains why changes in your daily habits, food, exercise, behaviours, environment and even your emotional state will make you more fertile (but can also make you less fertile). Knowing this will take you from a mindset of battling infertility to seeing it as a call to re-create your health and reprogramme your epigenome. I'm sharing this knowledge because it returns the power back to you. *You* are the only person who can change your circumstances, restoring your health to the best version it can be, regardless of the cards that you may have been dealt in life. You are capable of incredible change that can all come from within you. Even small changes – for example, eating lots of dark-green leafy vegetables – can make a big difference; they are rich in folate, which is vitally important for creating epigenetic tags on DNA, which control what happens to DNA and, ultimately, affects every cell and how it behaves. So something as simple as adding more vegetables to your diet can have major consequences for your fertility, and this knowledge makes these new habits easier to stick to.

Even if you haven't been following a lifestyle to optimize your health until now, most epigenetic changes are reversible. Though some of our epigenome is inherited (especially the one affecting our nervous system), an overwhelming amount is acquired, which means that we have direct control over it. Our bodies continually restructure, replenish and regenerate, and so you have the power to alter your body's destiny and take ownership of your own fertility.

Being in constant communication

Every minute of every day our bodies, and therefore our cells, are in a constant state of communication with our environment. Your body isn't one whole entity, but a collection of trillions of cells, according to the pioneering developmental biologist Dr Bruce Lipton. And each of those cells – including the DNA inside each one – will change according to its environment. This internal environment changes not only according to what we eat and how we exercise, as well as what we touch, breathe and taste, but also according to the state of our mind. Lipton says that if we feel loved, our blood will contain feel-good and vitality-enhancing hormones such as dopamine and oxytocin, as well as growth hormone. But if we feel fear, our blood becomes filled with stress hormones and inflammatory agents. In fact studies have shown that these changes in our blood can occur within the space of minutes. In Chapter 2 we'll look in greater depth into how your mind affects your body. Increasingly recent research is pointing to our cells as the main orchestrators of our destinies rather than our genes, and this is what's changing the narrative around our biology. Cells are capable of doing things that aren't necessarily written in our DNA – assuming roles and identities, exchanging information, creating and sculpting organs, sensing, learning and memorizing. To do what they need to, cells control which genes will be turned on or expressed, and so they decide where the products of the genes will be directed and used. Genes are not the architects, but merely tools that are used by cells to shape who we become.

What does this mean for your fertility?

It means that decisions we make regarding our health don't only impact upon us, but on the sperm and eggs from which our children will be formed, as well as the first environment they come into contact with: that of the womb. Investing in our health and lifestyle can literally shift the environment that supports our eggs and sperm, influencing their quality and their potential to give rise to healthy children.

How fast we age – including our eggs and sperm – is also an epigenetic process. And so how we live can even create an anti-ageing environment in the body that promotes sperm and egg health. This explains why some men and women over the age of forty are able to conceive naturally.

One way that ageing is kept in check is via an enzyme called telomerase. Its job is to replenish little caps on the end of DNA called telomeres, which preserve its integrity and structure. There are telomeres on the DNA in eggs and sperm. We know that telomerase is negatively affected by environmental factors such as poor diet, and by adverse events such as verbal or physical abuse, violence and trauma. However, the opposite is also true: love, compassion and support can enhance telomerase activity, thereby preserving telomeres and promoting health. This has been shown in patients with breast cancer.

When they joined a support group and practised regular meditation, they preserved their telomere lengths and curtailed the progress of disease. This strongly implies that we may be better able than we previously thought to alleviate the impact of ageing on eggs and sperm – even when, and how fast, egg and sperm quality starts to decline.

The implications for our children

The influence we can have on our genes doesn't start or end with us. It's *transgenerational*, meaning that our ancestors' behaviour and experiences have directly contributed to our own epigenome.

Some of this we can't control or influence. The experiences of our parents had a direct impact on our biological programming. But this also means that the choices we make in life will shape our children and the generations beyond. Becoming pregnant is one thing, but bringing a conscious awareness to the human being that is being shaped on the other side is another. We can take action towards not only conceiving, but towards creating the healthiest baby and future adult possible. And we can do this by optimizing the environment of the uterus. One way is via chemical messengers known as neurotransmitters and their receptors, which aren't only found in the mother's brain, but across her entire endometrium (uterine lining).

The foetal brain is continually constructing itself in the womb, creating 250,000 nerve cells per minute. The connections that form between these nerve cells continue developing after birth and even during adulthood, but the womb is the first environment where they are formed. And neurotransmitters do more than affect the nervous system of the baby; they influence everything from circadian rhythms, the cardiovascular and digestive systems, to how a child perceives pain over the course of their life.

Maternal health before pregnancy really matters – a fact being reinforced by numerous studies. For example, research has shown that the babies of anxious pregnant mothers have higher heart rates in the womb, which may have an effect on the babies' cardiovascular system later in life. If the mother experiences severe stress or trauma while pregnant, it has been shown this can directly impact on the foetal nervous system too. And maternal stress even has a major role in conditioning the health of the child, as it's been linked with greater behavioural problems, autism spectrum disorder, sleep disorders and an altered immune function and microbiome, as well as with a shorter lifespan.

Epi markers – switches controlling how genes are expressed during gestation and after birth – can be entirely different even in individuals with the same genetic make-up. This has been shown in identical twins who have identical genes but different epigenetic markers. Take the example of autism. Autism spectrum disorder has more than doubled in the last twenty years, with one in forty-four children now affected by it. If this was only controlled by genes, the risk of autism would be the same in identical twins. But in fact if one identical twin is autistic, the risk of the other one being autistic too is only 36 per cent. It appears that a good deal of autism isn't simply genetic, but is also epigenetic, down to a combination of stressors acting on DNA. And it's the non-shared environmental factors during or after birth, in particular before the age of four, that account for this, where the environment of one twin's brain may be different enough from the other to trigger the condition. Neuroplasticity refers to the brain's ability to adapt and reorganize its function in response to different experiences and environments, which means that there is far more control over improving brain health and function than was ever thought possible in the past. And this starts with the environment that the mother is exposed to.

Think of your legacy

Paternal health matters to baby's health too. One reason we know this is because of studies looking at the sons of fathers who had varied food supplies during the years leading up to puberty. The fathers who had had a surplus of food ended up having sons who had a greater risk of cardiovascular disease and diabetes . . . and this effect was also passed on to the son's male children. It even affected the epigenome of both the father's and the son's sperm, even though the sons were too young at the time to produce sperm of their own. Studies also show that male smoking, even before puberty and before men start producing sperm, led to them having sons with a higher BMI.

Most people only start to make better decisions about their health when they decide to try for a baby. But the process influencing our natural fertility and general reproductive health starts much earlier. In fact the egg that gave rise to us actually began life in our grandmother's womb, in the ovaries of our mother *in utero*. This means that the choices and behaviour of our grandmothers impacted not only on our mothers, but on us too. And whereas none of us was able to control or influence what happened to our grandparents and parents, we can change some of the adverse influences that we have inherited, starting now.

Is this why so many people find it hard to conceive?

Without a shadow of a doubt, there is a global issue concerning the reproductive potential of both men and women. And many of the causes (as well as the solutions) are likely to be epigenetic, with consequences that keep being passed down. Plus, there's an increasing incidence of conditions such as endometriosis, polycystic ovarian disease, premenstrual syndrome (PMS), fibroids, ovarian and breast cancer, as well as heavy and painful periods.

Sperm counts are at their lowest since records officially began. Sperm quality has halved in the last forty years, while the incidence of testicular cancer has grown, along with the risk of undescended testicles in young boys, as well as genitourinary abnormalities, leading experts to dub the phenomenon 'testicular dysgenesis syndrome'. One estimate is that 40–50 per cent of infertility, in a heterosexual relationship, is male-factor-related.

The evidence is clear: what we are exposed to, and the lifestyle choices we make, will affect our sperm or eggs, and probably the health and fertility of our children. The pillars of TCP are based on the fact that we can transform this with changes in diet, sleep and exercise patterns. And as the next few chapters explain, also by changing our thoughts and being curious about our deep inner beliefs and the patterns that exist within our relationships, including the most important one we have – with ourselves.

Epigenetics offers us a chance to connect with the incredible potential of our genes, while also being able to birth an upgraded version of ourselves that is healthier, fitter and more fertile. No doubt it is going to overhaul how we view health and evolve medicine, handing over the power to the individual. But I also believe that epigenetics will merge the world of science and spirit, helping us to understand the mind–body–spirit connection, the subject of the next two chapters.

Before a caterpillar can become a butterfly, it goes through a stage of transformation. New cells called 'imaginal cells' appear, which hold new patterns of DNA expression and so new potential for growth. These imaginal cells combine with the old cells, and this mix eventually gives rise to the new butterfly structure. You could say that we humans can do this too: by tapping into the power of our epigenome, we can emerge as new beings, stronger and ultimately healthier. One of the greatest gifts that the desire to become a parent gives us is the opportunity to reflect on our lives so far, then to do something differently. Understanding epigenetics shows us that we not only have the tools for self-empowerment, but also the blueprint for health and fertility within us. We can rewrite our epigenome through healthier actions and behaviours that support our well-being and our ability to conceive.

Children teach us to be present and patient with them; but, first, we need to be present and patient with ourselves. When we bring a conscious awareness to how all our decisions may impact upon our children, we are empowered to change for the better and, by doing this, give them the best future.

HOW THE OUTSIDE GETS INSIDE

Inside every cell there's a nucleus and, inside that, is DNA. You might imagine the nucleus was the brain of the cell, but according to developmental biologist Dr Bruce Lipton, it's the cell membrane that has the ultimate control over epigenetic changes to DNA. Cell membranes have receptors that communicate with the chemical and electrical signals in their surrounding environment, converting these into signals that affect the cell nucleus and the DNA. The membrane acts like the brain of the cell, with its own consciousness. It perceives the environment, reacts to it and stores those experiences. This means that our cells have plasticity – that is, they feel and respond to whatever is going on inside our bodies before it gets to affect our genes.

The cell membrane is the gatekeeper between the environment we don't see and the behaviour that results. It's the threshold between our DNA and what is shaping it. When we change our thought patterns, or what we eat, or how we exercise, the membrane decides how the cell responds and if there are adjustments in the way our DNA is expressed.

When we understand that we can control and harness the power of these receptors as much as medication, if not more, it enables us to appreciate how capable we are of creating fertility.

CHAPTER 2

Mind–body medicine

Delta, in her early thirties, suffered from terrible bouts of lower abdominal pain that meant she attended A&E several times. After many rounds of investigations, doctors still couldn't find a cause.

The next time she came to hospital she was referred to me, to look for a different root of her problem. I was able to reassure Delta that her pelvic ultrasound scan looked normal. We discussed her medication – a whole range of various drugs that she'd been pre-scribed, including laxatives to treat constipation and antivirals that she took whenever she experienced outbreaks of genital herpes.

I asked her how she was feeling. Delta told me that being crip-pled by the pain made her feel older than her years, that she had no control over her own body and was ashamed that she was experiencing genital herpes, which she felt others (including the medical profession) would judge her for. She'd withdrawn into herself and had stopped going out, because many of her friends couldn't understand quite how debilitating her pain was and blamed her for cancelling engagements at the last minute.

Delta said she'd never spoken about any of this before, and she went on to tell me about her childhood and how, growing up, she'd faced neglect and an absence of affection, which eventually led to her neglecting her own emotions and being afraid to voice her needs. She found any form of intimacy difficult to handle and noticed that she emotionally 'shut down' with partners. But she also observed resentment that would spill out as anger, some-times triggered by partners, when she often found herself having an out-of-body experience in order to be able to express what she needed to. The longer I spoke to Delta, the more it seemed to me that the pain was possibly being triggered by a combination of different factors interacting together, which wouldn't show up on any of the common tests she'd had: repressed emotions, a dysregulated nervous system that was sensitized to stress, an immune reaction that was primed for inflammation, and an imbalance in her gut microbiome as a consequence of all the medication she was on. Together, these were probably creating a perfect storm of chronic inflammation (see Chapter 8), which is the body's natural response to physical or chemical stress, but, when it's long-lasting or chronic, can lead to all kinds of dysfunction in the body.

I gently suggested to Delta that she should try counselling and some mind–body therapies to help her deal with the emotional aspects, as well as taking steps to help heal her gut; this meant coming off the laxatives and antivirals and using other, non-medicated means of help. Delta looked relieved. She told me that no one had ever viewed her condition in this multi-dimensional way and that she was going to act on my advice.

A couple of months later, Delta hadn't needed to go to A&E again. She only took the antivirals infrequently, as her genital-herpes outbreaks became far less frequent. She improved her diet and started taking probiotics. And she began seeing a counsellor as well as an acupuncturist. Her relationship with her partner improved and, most importantly of all, her relationship with herself became far more compassionate and healthier. She stopped viewing herself as the victim of her condition and instead took charge of her own well-being, in order to start thriving and feeling more in control of her own body.

Why everything is connected

Delta's story may seem strange: how can someone who comes into hospital with stomach pain possibly be helped by counselling? Western culture has taught us to view our bodies in terms of separate organ systems – the gut, the lungs, the heart, and so on. But the truth is that the body is multi-dimensional. It is influenced by a range of internal and external environmental factors, including our mind. All of us is interconnected: mind, body and spirit.

For example, if you have a problem with your period, you may not have considered the role that your diet or daily movement habits play in regulating your cycle, let alone that your stress or childhood experiences may be affecting it. But a woman's menstrual cycle is one of the most important indicators of fertility and well-being – it's even referred to as the fifth vital sign when it comes to overall health. It's no surprise that periods are interconnected with many other systems of the body and therefore act as a barometer of overall health.

Some of the factors that influence your periods range from your thyroid gland right through to sex-hormone imbalances, changes in weight, problems with insulin (the hormone prompted by blood sugar), disturbances to your gut microbiome or sleep patterns, as well as stress, negative thought patterns and emotions.

As an aside, this is why I have concerns about women taking hormonal contraceptives for prolonged periods of time. I often see women who have been on the pill for the majority of their adult life, then come off it as they want to conceive and find it hard to get pregnant. When coming off the pill, 20 per cent of women will take some time to restore their normal cycling and in some cases, especially when the pill has been started early in life, coming off it can reveal irregular or absent menstruation that was never noted before. Most women resume natural cycling within six to twelve months of stopping the pill, but the restoration of fertility can be a concern for many women, along with experiencing heavy periods and cramps, sometimes for the first time. As the pill takes over the normal mechanism of hormonal control and suppresses ovulation and normal hormonal fluctuation, it can take a little while for communication between the brain and the ovaries to be restored following its use, especially if it's been taken for a long time.

Many women have endocrine disturbances they aren't even aware of, and because the pill does such a good job of masking these, it's important to get in tune with your body, so that you have time to deal with, and sort out, any issues that may have long-term implications, such as infertility. If you started the pill purely for contraceptive purposes when you were younger, then it may be a good idea to come off it for a couple of months and see how your body responds, while using barrier contraception if you aren't actively looking to conceive then. There's more on cycle monitoring in the 12-week plan. This is the bigger context to fertility: different systems operating in synchronicity, communicating via a series of biological messengers, which are all influenced by how we eat, sleep and exercise, and the thoughts we ruminate over each day.

The approach of TCP to health and fertility – as you'll see in the next few chapters – is radical. It's not simply about 'eat this' or 'exercise like that', although food and movement are important. It's a plan to put you in charge of your own fertility. The idea is, as you read through these first chapters, you'll begin to see patterns in your own life that it may be helpful to change. Then, at the end of each chapter, I'll introduce the healing tools and habits that you'll be adopting during the 12-week plan.

This chapter is going to explain how your endocrine or hormone system interacts with your thoughts and emotions.

Body–mind communication

Let's start with the placebo effect. This is when a person's health appears to improve just by virtue of them believing it will, after taking what's effectively an inactive medical treatment, or placebo. This is often dismissed as being of little value, but in fact some studies have concluded that it can be as strong as taking a drug or even having surgery. I get really excited whenever I hear about what the placebo effect can do, as it demonstrates the tremendous power of the mind when we bring a different level of awareness.

It's also a concrete example of how the mind and body interact. The mind and body are always talking, via multiple kinds of messengers: chemicals such as hormones, neurotransmitters, neuropeptides and cytokines, as well as electrical nerve impulses. It used to be thought that the resulting messages mainly went one way, from the brain to the body. But it's now clear that a whole range of organs – including the gut, heart, ovaries and womb – make messenger chemicals that interact with the central nervous system. Scans have shown that pain triggers activity in the brain and across the body, but so does a strong memory of a painful experience: it's a two-way system.

As these messengers interacting with cell receptors also underpin the basis of human emotions, it means many of your organs are sensing and generating emotions of their own. For example, the neurotransmitter serotonin communicates emotions, desires, memories and thoughts, and it has receptors in the gut as well as the brain.

Cells themselves have a form of memory too. They can store a particular constellation of receptors from an experience or memory. This could be why organ recipients often report that they find themselves taking on some part of the personality of their organ donor. And why many women feel a visceral connection with their child during pregnancy and beyond, even when that child does not survive. During pregnancy, cells from the foetus actually enter the mother's bloodstream: this is called microchimerism. Mothers literally carry their babies in their hearts and minds for ever.

There's more: these foetal cells retain stem-cell properties, so that if a mother's organ (for instance, the heart) is injured through disease, the cells have been shown to migrate there to help repair it. When musician and broadcaster Myleene Klass found this out, she said it helped her find 'peace' after four miscarriages. 'It sends out all these little messages and helps with the organs, helps tweak whatever needs to be strengthened, and that DNA is left behind . . . They never leave you.'

After a miscarriage, one of my patients told me she was finding it difficult that the cry of someone else's child was enough to trigger her to produce milk. I explained that this was simply her emotions having a direct neurological and hormonal effect – an incredible example of her body remembering the experience of being a mother and expressing that through lactation.

Hormones, feelings and fertility

One of TCP's pillars is about dealing with stress, because its role in infertility is becoming increasingly clear. In clinic, I've seen how trying to conceive – especially after being diagnosed with a health condition, or being older than the average mum – can add a level of stress that can feel overwhelming. TCP looks at the influence that emotional health, including stress, has on your internal environment, the biological systems that shape your health, and what you can do to change that.

The central nervous system, including the brain, controls gene expression all over your body. So your mental and emotional well-being directly feeds into your epigenome, affecting the development of health or disease.

Added to that, hormones are particularly sensitive to emotions and thoughts, as well as to lifestyle changes. We spend a large proportion of our time thinking – on average, thirty-five years. And so the content of our thoughts and emotions drives our lives. What was your last thought before you picked up this book? Was it empowering or disempowering? What are your usual emotions and thoughts? At stressful times it's so easy to slip into negativity – I'm not enough; I'm not doing enough – or into criticizing yourself in some other way. When you do this, how does it make you feel?

As the way we think and feel has a knock-on effect on our hormones, it affects our fertility and, in particular, any condition involving the ovaries, uterus or testicles. The endocrine system is made up of numerous glands all over the body, which control all aspects of your health, from general well-being, your immune system and your menstrual cycle, to fertility. Hormones are the chemical messengers that run between various glands, shaping the behaviour of each cell they come into contact with. The endocrine system is always trying to come back to balance. And so, when there are any disturbances or abnormalities in the system, no matter how subtle, the hormonal consequences are amplified across the body.

One of the brain's jobs is to be the main overseer of the endocrine system, constantly intercepting, responding and sending hormonal signals. A good way to look at the endocrine system is as part of your body's hardware, with the brain as the software. When the software has a glitch, the system doesn't work properly. And, for most of us, this glitch is very often negative thought patterns, difficult emotions or stress.

These are some key parts of the brain–endocrine connection:

* **The hypothalamus** is the hormonal control centre, found in the brain. It interprets hormonal and other signals, and sends out messages to control sex organs, as well as the uterus and many other organs. This process is very sensitive to stress.

* **The hypothalamic–pituitary–gonadal (HPG) axis** oversees puberty, ovulation, fertility and menstruation. For example, the hypothalamus releases gonadotrophin-releasing hormone (GnRH), which acts on the pituitary to lead to the release of follicle-stimulating hormone (FSH) and luteinizing hormone (LH), which in turn act on the ovaries or the testicles, leading to the release of oestrogen and progesterone (and, to a small extent, testosterone) in the ovaries, and testosterone in the testicles. You can see how when one tiny part of this goes wrong, it can have big consequences. When the HPG is out of balance – for instance, with polycystic ovaries – there can be consequences that aren't restricted to fertility, which extend to someone's metabolism and cardiovascular function.

Feeling emotional

It's important to deal with unhelpful emotional thought patterns and stress before they can have knock-on negative effects in the endocrine system and other body systems, creating physical imbalances and, eventually, disease such as infertility. Healing, as you'll see in the chapters on trauma and stress, as well as in Part 3 of the book, involves exploring the emotional context to disease.

We need to start being brave and inquisitive about what our emotions are telling us. A first step is learning to recognize what emotions are coming up for you, where you feel them in your body, and to get curious about what they are telling you. That includes emotions that feel difficult or uncomfortable – the ones we consider negative. In fact, especially those emotions. By doing this, we bring what's usually subconscious into the conscious domain, and so gain wisdom about ourselves. During the 12-week plan you'll learn to check in with your feelings on a daily basis.

Our culture tells us that these emotions are unwanted because they get in the way of normal functioning. It also encourages labelling emotions as good or bad. But emotions in themselves are inherently neither; they are merely messengers that help direct us to the places we need to heal, and they almost always point to a much deeper source of that emotion. And so we tend to push down, avoid, cover up, deny or even drug these kinds of feelings. When we do this, we are missing a real opportunity for healing.

There are some emotional patterns that are associated with certain health conditions. Just as smoking or drinking too much is a risk factor for heart disease, so these emotional patterns lead to changes that predispose you to disease in a particular part of the body. This is an expanding field of science called psychoneuroimmunology, which explains how our psychology is related to our nervous and immune systems. All conditions have an underpinning subconscious personality that supports their development, and which manifests in the cells and tissues of a particular organ. For example, the condition of endometriosis involves cells similar to the lining of the womb being found in places where they don't belong. Just as they have disconnected from the original source, often the woman affected by this condition will also have learned to dissociate from her emotional trauma and pain as a coping strategy, in order to survive. Our personalities develop as a result of our life experiences and coping behaviours, some of which can be maladaptive or modelled by the rest of society. Many are the result of what happens to us, rather than being us, and new research shows that rather than being fixed or something we're born with, they're fluid and can change.

As you'll see in Part 3, infertility, endometriosis and PCOS are each associated with distinct emotional patterns. And many chronic diseases, including infertility, are associated with depression and anxiety. Looked at holistically, your emotional struggles may not only be the consequence of having infertility, but may also be one of its root causes. Realizing this within our societies will help us understand quite how important mental health is and will raise general awareness of the impact this can have on people's long-term health. But despite the circumstances you may have been exposed to, change is possible, and your mind can be used to assist you towards wellness and fertility. If we can recognize, feel, deal with and heal our emotional self, then we can transform our emotional pain and prevent it taking root in the physical.

Emotion at the cellular level

When we change our thought patterns, just as much as what we eat and how we exercise, our cells respond to this and alter their behaviour.

Bruce Lipton has written of how the stories we tell ourselves about the situations we experience can become internalized and affect the biological behaviour of cells. This includes negative thought patterns, which might come from being put down, teased, discriminated against or abused. When repeated over time, these can become embedded in different organs, including the brain.

When emotional pain is unresolved, unexpressed and unintegrated, it can start to create cellular shifts that move from health towards disease, including depression, post-traumatic stress disorder (PTSD) and anxiety, which in turn impacts on our fertility. Studies show that mental stress and negative thoughts can create inflammation in the body by changing cell behaviour, and that if these thought patterns are repeated, they can reactivate the inflammation, contributing to infertility. However, when soothing techniques such as meditation and listening to music take place, they can help counteract inflammation with the relaxation response.

This kind of change is proof that you're not the victim of circumstances, or the cards you've been dealt genetically. You have far more power than you realize in being able to control the environment that you create for your cells to exist in.

Claiming this power back is what holistic medicine is all about. Just by thinking about your mind and body in a new way, you have begun to treat and manage the mental and spiritual components of fertility, rather than simply the physical dimension. You are a living, breathing matrix of energetic and chemical systems, able to influence your health by changing your environment and your physical body, but also through the power of your mind and (the subject of the next chapter) your spiritual life force.

Techniques you'll use to connect mind–body

Here are two of the tools you'll be using during the 12-week plan to bring greater awareness to the mind–body connection.

Visualization

One reason visualization works is that a belief about what you expect to happen sends instructions to the mind and body to start a chain of events that are the same as if the experience you visualized was actually happening, which leads to the expectation coming true. For example, research has found that imagining the act of lifting can lead to changes in muscle strength that can be measured.

Another reason it works is that imagining or recalling an act of kindness has been shown to have positive physiological effects. One route is via the activation of oxytocin, the love or kindness hormone. Kindness and compassion also activate the vagus nerve, the main nerve of the parasympathetic (rest-and-digest part of the) nervous system.

Visualization has been shown to help healing too. For instance, after a stroke, it can be used to repair damaged parts of the brain. And in a study of breast-cancer patients, those who practised visualization of their immune system effectively dealing with the cancer showed much greater activity of the immune system. As the mind and body intersect at the level of the imagination, remembering that our cells respond to emotion can help us understand how our nervous, immune and endocrine systems can be stimulated to act as if you were pregnant, through the act of visualization. I'll take you through this in Part 2 of the book.

Affirmations

Positive affirmations are a form of repetitive visualization that reinforce positive perspectives of our situation. They aren't just words; they rewire our brains and nervous system, which then creates biological change at the cellular level. Through affirmations we can expand our sense of self and diminish the threat of a problem or challenge. Combining loving compassion – where you practise speaking kindly to yourself – and positive affirmations may be of benefit when you're wanting to conceive. Several of my patients have told me it has helped them to speak affirmations out loud to themselves or to write them down in a journal. However, don't confuse positive affirmations with ignoring or painting over difficult emotions. It's vital that these feelings are addressed and processed, rather than denied, in addition to using affirmations to help change your perspective.

CHAPTER 3

Going deeper: emotions and energies

When it comes to infertility, alternative therapies are often people's place of last resort. In clinic, someone will often say, 'Well, nothing else seemed to work, so we thought we may as well give it a go.' Then, when they go on to benefit from these treatments, they tell me they wish they'd done them sooner!

In the UK one in six of us now engages in alternative therapies such as acupuncture, reflexology and mind–body treatments. There is greater recognition of the usefulness of these therapies in clinical scenarios too: in the US, this is one function of the National Center for Complementary and Integrative Health.

Alternative therapies are a fundamental part of TCP. Working at the level of energy, they take TCP's holistic approach to fertility even deeper. In my experience, the best approach to preconception (and to overall health too) considers the whole person. And ancient medicine systems such as Chinese medicine and Ayurveda have a long history of treating all the components of a patient: the physical, mental, emotional and spiritual.

Conception is undeniably a spiritual process. One of my patients described it as something that's so much bigger than us, where we realize there is a flow of energies beyond our humanness waiting to be discovered and connecting us all with the Universe. The spiritual element of not getting pregnant also has a deeper meaning, leading you to evolve past who you are now and to embody the attributes that help to restore your wholeness (the word 'whole' refers to healing, which means that wholeness is a consequence of healing). So the question you might ask yourself is, 'What is not getting pregnant trying to get me to heal and learn about myself?' Becoming a parent is first and foremost a spiritual assignment. A vital element of TCP is about taking care of your spiritual needs and, in the process, discovering a new version of yourself. Once you've done that, a natural consequence will be that you're not only improving your chances of conceiving, but you're in a much better position to birth another human being, bringing a whole new level of consciousness to parenting.

One of the reasons alternative therapies can be so effective is that they lead to upgrades in consciousness, not just in the mind but, more importantly, in the cells of our body, each of which has its own consciousness too. We know this through work that has been done on the cell membrane, showing that it acts like a second brain in the cell (see Chapter 1).

Western medicine, for all its incredible advances and technologies, has excelled when it comes to treating acute disease, but there's been far less progress when it comes to chronic disease, such as endometriosis, PCOS and, of course, infertility. Despite improvements in assisted reproductive techniques, such as IVF, success rates aren't much above 50 per cent at best. There is still a high rate of 'unexplained' infertility, where IVF is often encouraged, but in the absence of identifying or treating the underlying problems, it can be akin to a sticking-plaster approach, rather than dealing with the root causes.

As a doctor, I want to maximize the benefits that I can deliver to my patients, which means taking a holistic approach. Although we may not yet have studies and data on holistic therapies that are robust enough to appease some sceptics, this is not a reason to dismiss them. As I've seen in clinic, sometimes these treatments are what is needed, alongside conventional medicine, instead of more invasive therapies, because they make the most of the body's own natural healing capacity.

The energy–spirit–healing connection

There is now consensus that an energetic system exists not only in the body, but surrounding it too. Every biological organism – including you and me – has a biofield. It's made up of an electromagnetic field that comes from the various electrical and magnetic charges that move within and outside the bodily system, as well as small particles of light. It can be scientifically measured and recorded by an EEG (an electroencephalogram, a recording of brain activity) or MRI (magnetic resonance imaging, a scan of the body). This energetic body system can influence your physical body, including cell behaviour and hormonal processes within it. It's been shown that our cells are capable of generating light (not detectable to the naked eye) and an electromagnetic field as a means of communicating with each other and with our external biofield, like antennae constantly sending and receiving information. As medical doctor and thought leader Zach Bush explains, our bodies can be seen as solar events existing in particle states.

The biofield is sometimes also called the auric field or aura. It's like another sense with which we can experience the world – a sixth sense. Although alternative therapies have a variety of heritages, most of them have the same approach: healing via the body's energetic systems. Some therapies are also biologically based (supplements, herbs and diet); others are body-based (chiropractic, massage); some are mind-based (counselling, hypnosis); mind–body based (yoga, meditation, mindfulness); or a combination of these (acupuncture, Ayurveda). Some are predominantly energetically based (reiki, crystal healing). But, ultimately, they all interact with the biofield.

Your body is always trying to balance the energetic and chemical input from your environment and from inside of you, with your cells and organs constantly communicating on this. Health or disease is a natural side-effect of this attempt to reach a state of balance. Symptoms, such as pain or an abnormal menstrual bleeding pattern, can be calls to action, sending important messages that we need to get back into balance.

Alternative therapies can help realign distorted energetic patterns and, by doing so, boost our natural biological healing process. Perhaps it's better to call them complementary therapies, because they complement the natural biological processes and include the mind as a vital part of their approach.

How emotion and energy link

There is another way to heal energies: by healing your emotions. The previous chapter looked at how our emotions and thoughts influence the entire internal environment that shapes our health, via our cells and our biological systems. They do this through your mind, your physical body and your energetic body. We talked about how emotional patterns that lead to health conditions such as infertility can be rooted in past adverse experiences or trauma (more on this in the next chapter too).

Disease, more often than not, has its roots in the emotional plane. Mental and emotional energies, thoughts and feelings can become physical, either through the bodily chemicals they generate, such as hormones, or through the frequencies associated with their vibration.

The holistic approach to health and fertility, which embraces this energetic model, turns a lot of conventional medicine on its head, because rather than disease coming from internal dysfunction in a cell or an organ, it suggests that disease is due to states of consciousness that create energetic imbalances that translate down to the physical level and influence cell behaviour. This is the psycho-physical model of health and disease. Many alternative practitioners believe that even before a disease manifests, it may show up in the biofield of a patient, suggesting several points for intervention before something has had a chance to become a disease. This idea of fertility being a feature of something going on outside our physical selves is reinforced when we look at the initial development of an embryo, and the fact that the cells that will make up the reproductive tract actually infiltrate from the outside – something referred to as the yolk sac, which is attached to the embryo. The outside eventually manifests on the inside. When we process emotion and integrate experiences, we allow an energetic shift to happen that affects our biofield, which leads to a change in consciousness affecting our minds and our cells, which ultimately leads to a change in the physical body.

Routes into healing the energetic body

The meridian system

The meridian system comes from ancient Chinese medicine. Meridian lines are the lines of energetic flow between various organs, alongside the blood and lymph systems. In Chinese medicine this system is accessed through acupuncture points; acupuncturists and energetic healers have been using this system to heal for many thousands of years. It's a way that your mind and emotions connect with the physical body and with the energetic and spiritual body. Some of the therapies you will be doing in the 12-week plan will help you access these meridians.

The meridians develop before any other system in the body, just fifteen hours after conception, making it the most primal method of communication between our cells and tissues. Meridian fluid follows the path of meridian lines, carrying bioenergetic and biochemical information that can shape the epigenome around the body. And meridians are important in organ and cell regeneration. The fluid provides a blueprint that influences what happens to a particular organ and, when the flow of meridian fluid is obstructed, it affects the health of the tissues.

The chakras

Accessing the chakras can be a powerful way to improve your fertility. You'll be doing this during the 12-week plan through specific chakra meditations. There are seven main chakras. You could describe them as the organs of the energetic system. They are points where information flows between the physical body and the energetic body. They are situated in a line down the centre of your body, going from the root chakra at the base of your spine, up to the crown chakra at the top of your head.

The chakras act as conductors of information and process energetic input too. They are constantly transforming and distributing emotional signals to various parts of the body, linking our energetic body with our physical body and expressing either health or disease.

The chakras communicate by means of their own non-physical series of energetic channels called nadis, which are supported by the meridian system. Like the meridians, nadis are formed very soon after conception. But while the meridians follow the blood system around the body, the nadis follow the distribution of the nervous system and are linked to the endocrine system. Chakras are always communicating between one another. A dysfunction at the level of one will affect the others and will translate to a hormonal disturbance. This is one of the reasons why looking at fertility always means that we have to look at what else is happening in the rest of the body too.

The reverse is also true: once you start to work on one chakra, you affect them all. This is the beauty of holistic medicine; it's about creating space for treating and managing the mental and spiritual components of infertility, as well as the physical ones, where each has a knock-on effect on the others, as they're all closely and inextricably intertwined.

7 MAIN CHAKRAS

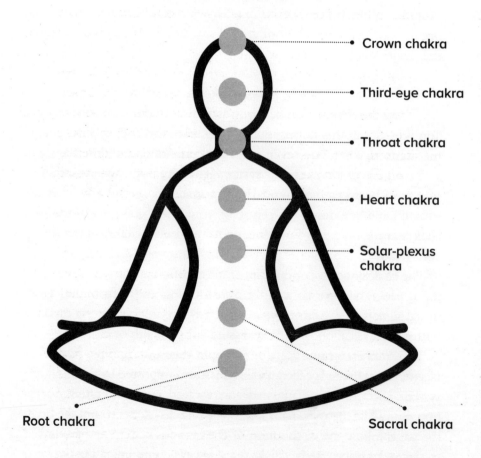

A HEALING GUIDE TO USING THE CHAKRAS

Each chakra influences particular organ systems and emotions. Blockages can show up as emotional and/or physical problems.

Root chakra

Linked to survival, the root chakra is associated with the pelvic organs as well as the adrenal glands and the stress response. It's connected to childhood emotions around trust, belonging and boundaries, as well as issues relating to being accepted. Dysfunction can show up as co-dependency, self-sabotage and issues around trust.

Sacral chakra

This chakra is related to the reproductive organs, relationships and the ability to express our sexuality. It's linked to trauma from abuse, exploitation, betrayal and sexual wounding, and to our relationship with our mother. Blocks show up as problems in the cervix, uterus and ovaries, as well as abandonment, shame, insecurity, fear over being true to yourself, and ambiguity around having children.

Solar-plexus chakra

The solar-plexus chakra is linked to power, which goes back to childhood and how your experiences shaped the lens through which you now perceive the world. If many of your needs as a child were never met, it's likely that you grew up feeling unsafe to fully express yourself in the world. These inner-child issues can leave people feeling they have little or no control over their lives. Emotional imbalances include anger, a sense of overwhelm, dependency and passivity, as well as a lack of self-worth. Dysfunction here can make us more sensitive to stress and cause digestive problems, such as ulcers, IBS (irritable bowel syndrome) or inflammatory bowel disease.

Heart chakra

This is where love towards the self and others is expressed. If we were never taught or given permission to meet our own needs, this can lead to self-depletion and self-sacrifice and eventually to resentment. It's also associated with grief and depression. The heart chakra is linked to heart and breast problems, but also to immune conditions, endometriosis and premature ovarian ageing. Often considered the most important chakra, it's the gateway between the upper and lower chakras. This is why going into our hearts during meditation is so important.

Throat chakra

The portal of communication, the throat chakra is associated with the thyroid, mouth and parasympathetic (rest-and-digest) nervous system. It's closely linked with the vagus nerve that connects the brainstem with the heart, lungs and abdominal organs. Blocks lead to a feeling of not being heard and an inability to express our truth, which leads to suppression of our needs and subservience.

Third-eye or brow chakra

Also known as the seat of our intuition, the third eye is connected to the pineal gland as well as the eyes, ears, nose, sinuses and spinal cord. As this centre also has an association with the pituitary gland, one of the major endocrine organs, imbalances in this area can lead to a range of hormonal disturbances.

Crown chakra

A psychic centre of perception, the crown chakra is concerned with the spiritual essence of who we are and has close links with the spiritual body. It's related to the cerebral cortex or higher brain. If there is dysfunction, it can lead to overwhelm and confusion. When balanced, this chakra opens us up to a multitude of other sensory inputs beyond our mere physical senses.

Alternative therapies to try

Think of these therapies as an investment in your well-being. These treatments are not fast fixes. They usually work best in combination and over a longer period of time – at least three months prior to conception. There are some for which you may wish to see a practitioner, and others that you can learn the basic techniques of to help yourself (these are in the 12-week guide, see page 198). They may often release deep-seated emotions, so I encourage you to consider psychological support from a counsellor, who can help you work through what arises for you.

* **Reiki**: the practitioner moves energies around you, restoring flow and communication between the different energetic centres. Reiki activates the parasympathetic nervous system, helping to reduce the impact of stress. In a study looking at pain and anxiety levels in women who had abdominal hysterectomies, those who received reiki alongside conventional treatment had lower pain and anxiety scores and needed fewer painkillers.

* **Osteopathy**: a hands-on approach to relieving restrictions and pain. As the central nervous system is connected to surrounding organs through connective tissue called fascia, relieving the tension here can help to calm you. In patients with endometriosis, who often have considerable pelvic-floor tension, a study showed that osteopathic treatment led to 80 per cent having physical improvement of their symptoms, and 70 per cent experiencing psychological relief.

* **Chiropractic therapy**: treating pinched or pressed nerves as well as spinal distortions caused by accidents, illnesses

or stress. Chiropractic can help for similar reasons to osteopathy, but in particular it can focus on the spinal cord, the central highway of nerves. There are studies reporting an increase in pregnancies following chiropractic care. A technique called 'network spinal analysis' helps the nervous system to form better connections with organs, including those of the reproductive system, releasing tension created by trauma. Kinesiology is a similar form of treatment, combining muscle-testing with Traditional Chinese Medicine in order to gain insights into areas of stress and imbalance in the biofield and the central nervous system.

❊ **Shamanism**: shamans were the original neuroscientists of ancient civilizations, and they understand how to work on the energetic and spiritual body to bring old pain and trauma to consciousness and release it. Research shows that shamanic healing methods, such as drumming and chanting, can produce a profound healing and reorganizing effect on the brain that is similar to psychedelics.

❊ **Acupuncture and acupressure**: stimulation of specific points in the body with needles, pressure, suction (cupping) or electrical stimulation. Chinese medicine says there are more than 2,000 of these points, connected via meridians and nadis. Stimulation can help to reduce pain as well as inflammation and may also help to balance hormones, regulate ovulation and increase blood flow to the reproductive organs. These therapies are now NHS treatment options for chronic pain. Studies have shown they can improve the number of mature eggs collected during fertility treatment.

❊ **Hypnotherapy**: this involves reaching a state of deep relaxation via the guidance of a hypnotherapist, whereby you're able to tap into the subconscious part of your brain, where your thoughts, beliefs, emotions and memories originate, so that they can be processed, to drive more health-enhancing behaviour. Studies have shown that hypnosis can help to improve the success of embryo transfer during an IVF cycle.

✳ **Sound therapy**: using the sound vibrations of gongs, tuning forks, drums, sound bowls and ultrasound to bring the body back into balance. It is good for stress reduction, as demonstrated by a study done by the British Academy of Sound Therapy, which showed that it turned down the autonomic (fight-or-flight) nervous system. It's also been shown to help increase the chance of pregnancy and reduce inflammation, as well as improve blood flow to the reproductive organs.

✳ **Fertility astrology and Human Design/Gene Keys**: these therapies draw on astrology, the I Ching, the Kabbalah and the chakra system to explain how each of us is uniquely hardwired and how to live in alignment. It also looks at our core wounds and patterns, some of which we've inherited and others we've sustained over this lifetime (many of which contribute to our epigenome), to enable us to draw a deeper connection with our inner truth and embody the consciousness of our lessons. Astrological medicine also believes that the zodiac is topographically represented within our bodies, with each zodiac sign corresponding to a different organ system.

✳ **Biofield therapy**: this describes various techniques that work with the biofield of the body to help release and process emotions and integrate trauma in order to create a regenerated biofield. It includes treatments such as Healing Touch, Transference Healing and chakra balancing, to name just a few. It's also believed that this form of treatment may help to create a receptive space for an incoming soul to enter and integrate. As a relatively new form of healing, research on biofield therapy is scarce, but there are case-study reports of positive effects on fertility and pregnancy.

CRYSTAL THERAPY

Crystal healing is thought to come from the Earth's geo-magnetic field interacting with our human biofield. Each crystal has its own electromagnetic properties and geo-metric patterns that occurred through the solidification of minerals over time, giving it frequencies that can be used to influence our energetic body. Certain colours of crystals resonate with particular emotions and their associated chakras too. Crystals can also be used as your point of focus during meditation. I'll suggest some crystals to use for different emotions in the 12-week plan.

A NOTE ON HOMEOPATHY

Homeopathy views symptoms as messages and calls to action, and rather than taking a suppressive approach, it explores the emotional basis behind disease and adopts a mutli-dimensional view that takes the mind, body and spirit all into account, as well as the energetic body. It operates on the basis that disease, such as infertility, is due to an imbalance in vital force and seeks to create a rebalance through the principle of treating like with like, and empowering the individual to heal themselves. Tiny amounts of natural substances, such as plants and minerals, are used to stimulate the healing process. Studies have shown that homeopathy can help with both male and female factor infertility.

CHAPTER 4

Infertility

If you are reading this book because you have already been trying to get pregnant, but it hasn't yet happened, this chapter is for you. It outlines some of the theories and causes of infertility, as well as ways to take positive, holistic ownership of your mindset and your reproductive health and journey towards becoming a parent.

Infertility remains one of the most elusive conditions to treat. It's not even recognized as a disease by many people. It's also the only area of medicine where a diagnosis of 'unexplained' has become widely accepted. 'Unexplained' means that the usual tests (see page 50) can't offer a reason as to why a couple isn't getting pregnant.

Research shows that up to one-third of infertility is classified as unexplained. For the rest, ovulatory disorders (the commonest of these being polycystic ovaries), male-factor infertility (which is estimated to be a contributing factor in up to almost half of all cases), tubal abnormalities, such as scarring, and endometriosis are among the most common causes.

Why is there so much infertility that appears unexplained? One of the commonest and most obvious answers is that people tend to be older when they start trying for children now, compared to previous generations. More than half are now child-free at thirty, for the first time since records began. And, without doubt, age does influence fertility. But there's more to it, because globally, fertility levels are in decline, even among the younger generations. This is the consequence of an environment that is no longer conducive to becoming pregnant – including our exposure to toxins, lack of sleep, stress levels as well as our disconnect in relationships and with ourselves.

The idea of TCP is to help you find all the factors that could be contributing to you not getting, or staying, pregnant. But there are some factors, primarily emotional patterns, that traditional medicine either ignores or minimizes, but which are just as important and which we'll also explore in this chapter. It's not merely down to age; even if you are over forty, there is a lot you can still do to optimize your chances of conceiving. Your job now is to work on as many of these suggestions as possible.

The infertility pathway: a practical guide

If you've been trying to get pregnant for a year if you're thirty-five and under (or six months if you're over thirty-five), or if you have a reason to be concerned about your fertility (such as a previous diagnosis of endometriosis or a sexually transmitted disease, or STD), see your GP. These are some of the standard fertility investigations you may be offered.

* **Blood tests**: a progesterone test done on Day 21 for a regular 28-day menstrual cycle (day of the test varies, depending on cycle length). Also an FSH test and often LH too, early in your menstrual cycle. This can also offer useful information on ovarian (egg) reserve. (Another hormone tested for ovarian reserve is anti-Müllerian hormone, or AMH, but most GPs don't provide this test.) Your GP may also test for thyroid hormones and for the hormone prolactin, both of which can affect fertility.

* **STD screening**

* **Ultrasound**: a referral for a transvaginal ultrasound scan to look at your pelvis for any abnormalities, and to assess your ovaries and your womb. Ideally during this scan the number of follicles, or small fluid-filled sacs containing your egg cells, should be counted to give an indication of your ovarian reserve.

* **Fallopian tube test**: if you have a positive STD screening or a previous history of STDs, or a condition such as

endometriosis, or if there are signs of abnormalities affecting your Fallopian tubes on a previous scan, you may be offered a test to check if the tubes are open. Hysterosalpingo-Contrast Sonography (HyCoSy) uses ultrasound and dye, while Hysterosalpingography (HSG) uses X-ray and dye.

* **Sperm analysis**: to look at volume, concentration, motility (movement) and morphology (shape) of the sperm.

If your GP then refers you to a specialist, you may be offered:

* **Laparoscopy or keyhole surgery**: if you've had pelvic inflammatory disease (PID) in the past, or there's an indication that you may have abnormalities affecting your Fallopian tubes, or if you have a large ovarian cyst or if it's suspected that you may have endometriosis.

* **Hysteroscopy**: a camera is passed into the womb to assess the inside of it. Anything that might be interfering with pregnancy, such as scar tissue, polyps or smaller fibroids, can be removed. (If you have fibroids, depending on their location and size, you may be referred for a bigger operation.)

After any procedures, you may be advised to continue trying naturally or to have fertility treatment (see Chapter 14).

What is secondary Infertility?

This is a problem in becoming pregnant after you have conceived at least once before. People often underestimate how common it is. In fact it's the most common type of infertility among women.

Aside from the effect of age and the impact this has on egg numbers and quality, secondary infertility may be due to the onset or progression of medical or gynaecological conditions, such as fibroids, endometriosis or Asherman's syndrome (scar tissue in the womb).

Your lifestyle habits may also have changed and your partner's sperm may not quite be what it used to be, or you may have a new partner whose fertility is different.

Many couples in this situation are hesitant about seeking help, worrying about feeling judged by others, including their doctor, especially if they already have a child. But the advice remains the same as it is for primary infertility: if you've been trying for a year if you're thirty-five and under, or six months if you're over thirty-five, see your GP to start some initial investigations.

IVF: too fast a fix?

Assisted reproductive technologies (ARTs), such as IUI (intrauterine insemination), IVF, egg-freezing and donation (see Chapter 14), exist to help people with fertility. They enable more people than ever before the opportunity to become a parent. However, doctors often advise patients – including those with unexplained infertility – to go straight for IVF, assuming it will save them time and money. Sadly, IVF is not a magic formula or a pill to fix infertility. Conception rates remain low, in particular in those aged over forty, despite IVF being available.

Even so, many fertility clinics don't offer enough of an exploration into the causes of infertility, or support more natural routes to conception where possible, or advise on ways to optimize the epi markers before having IVF or another form of ART. Sometimes it's only later down the line, when a few attempts with IVF haven't been successful, that you might be offered further physical investigations. And mind–body techniques are often reserved as a last resort.

The problem is that it's difficult to move forward when you can't understand the root causes contributing to why you're not getting pregnant. As the attempts at IVF rack up, your mental health can suffer. While IVF may have seemed like a fast fix at first, in many cases it's far from it and can ultimately leave you feeling disempowered.

By reducing conception to a mechanical process, ART can miss vital pieces of the puzzle that make up someone's fertility. Fertile health is a complex interaction between the endocrine, neurological and immune systems, along with the emotions, psychology and general health. Doing TCP may sidestep the need for IVF, but if it doesn't, it will create the optimum conditions for IVF success, if that is the route you end up going down. It will teach you to seek for answers inside you, rather than outside, which returns the power to you.

Emotions: cause or consequence?

Trying to get pregnant is stressful, which is why one of the pillars of TCP is a focus on stress. And the longer the wait for pregnancy, the more the distress will grow. People say that being told to 'just relax' by well-intentioned, though not necessarily well-informed friends and family is the single most frustrating piece of advice they get given. Psychological distress due to infertility is often dismissed as inevitable. Most medical professionals focus only on the physical elements and don't acknowledge the bigger emotional context of this condition.

But 75 per cent of people who are struggling to get pregnant have anxiety and/or depression. And infertility has all the hallmarks of trauma, just as many other medical diseases do. As the psychologist Allyson Bradow points out, trauma involves the psychological and emotional response not only to physical threats, but also to deeply held expectations of life, of which childbearing is one of the most important ones.

Being exposed to persistent reminders of this expectation by family, friends and colleagues, as well as interactions with those who are pregnant, means that if you are struggling with infertility you are constantly triggered by what you don't have.

We need to think about infertility as a chronic disease – one that's almost as common as cancer. Governments don't consider not having children to be life-threatening, which is why there hasn't been enough investment towards diagnosis or cure, and why most people have to fund treatment themselves.

Because there is little awareness of the emotional stress of infertility, and because feelings of grief or anguish are not necessarily 'allowed', it's common to repress these emotions. As you'll see in Chapter 5, this is important and can have significant long-term consequences because of what we now understand about how unprocessed emotions can impact on our bodies, including our fertility, but also on the health of our future children.

The importance of feeling your emotions

You may be finding your emotions hard to bear, but in fact they are useful. Think of them simply as messengers, signals to capture your attention and tell you about your inner environment. They translate the language of your nervous and endocrine systems and give a reading of what's going on at the level of your cells, so that you can become more self-aware and take action.

But because we've been conditioned to avoid painful feelings, we don't stop to consider the intelligence and wisdom contained in them. Instead we develop coping behaviours that keep us detached from our emotions, without experiencing their full impact. And sometimes that coping behaviour can take the form of further rounds of IVF, or carrying on trying, without necessarily giving yourself time to process your feelings, because even the thought of pausing feels too painful.

As well as stress, one of the other most common patterns that I see with infertility is sexual disharmony, which is covered in Chapter 10. I also see a lot of unprocessed grief, as well as a whole host of other difficult emotions, such as envy, disappointment and shame. On top of that, I often witness a disconnect between what the person is expressing and what they are feeling.

Remember, all these feelings are normal and deeply human. Recognizing them, and perhaps also knowing that other people with similar experiences are dealing with them too, will start moving them through you. It's important to take time to process emotions, ideally before you become pregnant, and it's important to seek help in being able to do this. This is especially true if trying to get pregnant has been taking a long time, which can compound the trauma. Opening yourself up to emotions takes courage and vulnerability, but it also opens the door to transformation and healing at both an emotional and a physical level. 'Feel it to heal it,' as they say.

WATCH OUT FOR LANGUAGE

Infertility is a place where language really matters. Anyone who's ever experienced the loss of or dream of a baby will tell you they remember every single aspect of it, from the smell of the doctor's office to the look in the nurse's eyes, but especially the words spoken to them.

During fertility treatment there is repeated use of the word 'fail': failed cycle, failed transfer, failed egg collection, failed fertilization and failed insemination. This reflects the toxic belief that becoming pregnant is about aggressive pursuit, rather than an act of going inwards and surrendering to the messages that your body is communicating, as well as listening to your feelings.

Or think of the word 'miscarriage'. It seems to imply that someone did something wrong in carrying their baby. Or a 'chemical pregnancy'. That term can be upsetting, suggesting something that is not there, but should have been. Even the word 'infertility' sounds bleak and sterile, conjuring up notions of inadequacy. Medical vocabulary lacks sensitivity, referring to babies who were lost too soon as 'products of conception', 'foetal remains' or a 'blighted ovum'. Or to women's cervixes as 'incompetent'. The language needs to change. Until then, if you can be aware of its inadequacy, it may help you stop going down the emotional rabbit hole of self-blame, judgement, criticism and self-loathing.

Triggers and traits

Even if you have a chronic condition that impacts on fertility, such as endometriosis or PCOS, there may also be emotional factors underlying that. In addition, there are certain personality traits that seem to be more prevalent in people with infertility. For women, these are covered in Part 3, in the chapters relating to particular conditions. Men who suffer from infertility tend to have lower self-esteem, social assertiveness and are more withdrawn. It's easy to assume these traits are due to the person suffering from infertility. But it's also possible that they suggest certain emotional states or patterns of dysfunction that might in themselves be contributing to infertility. New research has shown that certain personality traits are associated with being at risk for chronic health conditions.

Exploring these issues is a vital part of being able to understand what could lie behind your struggle to conceive. Support for this should be one of the first steps before more invasive treatment, such as ART. This may require the help of a counsellor or therapist. An increasing number of studies are beginning to show the positive effect of psychotherapy and mind–body–spirit work in improving pregnancy rates for those with infertility, especially those who require ART. The 12-week plan includes self-exploration into these areas too. This is really worth doing. After all, children will be our biggest triggers and teachers in life. Doing the work *before* we become pregnant means that we will be better parents and will cultivate better and more insightful relationships with our children. Ultimately, it will liberate our children from the unhelpful and sometimes damaging emotional patterns that can affect us.

CHAPTER 5

Healing trauma, feeling whole

Annie was in her mid-thirties and was suffering from mild endometriosis. She and her partner had attempted to conceive naturally for almost two years, without success.

Even as she came into the consulting room with her husband, she began telling me that there was nothing I could do for them, aside from providing IVF – something they weren't keen on. 'I didn't even see the point in coming to the appointment. You're just going to tell me what I've heard before. We might as well save ourselves the time and effort.' She presented herself as though she had made peace with her situation. But behind this veneer, what I saw was someone who was deeply wounded and vulnerable, her trauma hidden behind a wall of defensiveness, which was also keeping her detached from the pain of facing her own feelings.

As we talked, we got on to the subject of birth. I asked Annie, if she were to become pregnant, whether she'd considered how she would give birth. Immediately she said, 'By Caesarean of course!' That she was so emphatic struck me, so I asked her to explain. With her arms and legs crossed, she told me that her mother often said that if Annie had her own baby, she'd have to have a Caesarean because it was the only safe form of birthing. Her mother had also advised her to think twice about whether she really wanted to have a baby at all.

Annie's mother had given this advice with the best of intentions. But Annie had ended up internalizing her mother's own traumatic birth experience and her resulting views. The message her body had received was that it wasn't safe to become pregnant. And so it made sense that Annie's body would protect her, by preventing her from becoming pregnant, just as she was trying to protect herself from feeling her own vulnerabilities through defensiveness and a disconnect with her real emotions. I suspected that this internalized trauma, as well as Annie's current anxieties, was also contributing to the flare-ups of her endometriosis.

I asked Annie and her husband what they wanted to do. They said they simply couldn't see themselves getting pregnant naturally, so they wanted to proceed to IVF.

I said, 'Can I be honest?' I really wasn't sure how what I was about to say would be received. They both nodded. I said to Annie, 'I believe you're not getting pregnant because I think you're terrified. You may not realize you are, but your entire body feels scared to conceive.'

I paused. Maybe Annie wasn't ready to hear this. Perhaps she might think it was not my place to tell her. Instead she turned and reached out to her husband and began to cry.

Annie said that no one had ever said this to her before, but she knew it was true and it felt like a relief to admit it. In that moment she gave herself permission to experience all her feelings, instead of putting on a brave face. We talked about what might help, including counselling. And I asked them to return in six months if they were still struggling to conceive naturally. I also asked Annie to do some work with a healer, to deal with the impact of the birth trauma that she was brought into the world with.

Annie started seeing a counsellor who worked on her being able to view pregnancy as a positive, safe experience, no matter how she decided to birth her future baby. She also saw a shaman and a chiropractor, who helped her to deal with her early-life trauma and the effect on her nervous system, as well as an acupuncturist. She found that her relationship with her husband improved, and her endometriosis-related pain was significantly alleviated and became less frequent. Within six months Annie became pregnant naturally. With support through her antenatal journey, she gave birth, vaginally, to a healthy baby girl.

We tend to associate trauma with people who've been through significant life-changing events – for example, army veterans or people who've survived life-threatening circumstances. But in fact trauma affects all of us, and usually from a young age. Whether it's losing a beloved pet, experiencing your family breaking up, poverty, racism, suffering emotional abuse or living in a war zone, trauma has no boundaries or hierarchies.

Trauma doesn't have to come from an 'event'. It can arise from our family dynamics and cultural beliefs, as well as from the way society treats us. The stories we come to embody from a young age, the adversities we've experienced or the beliefs we've internalized become the defining storylines of our life. That is, until we see that they're really the residue of previous trauma, which shapes the lens through which we experience the world, and our minds and bodies too. Infertility, itself a traumatic situation, can reveal the place where healing needs to occur at a deep level, often connecting us back to some form of trauma from the earlier days of our life.

This chapter looks at where your trauma might have come from, and helps you explore how it might have affected your fertility. Trauma isn't so much about what exactly happened to us. Rather, it's the response to circumstances that felt overwhelming or threatening at the time. Gabor Maté, a doctor and author specializing in trauma, describes it as 'a normal response to abnormal situations'. And the reason this is so relevant to fertility is that trauma can become ingrained in our bodies and our nervous system, contributing to disease.

Most of us haven't been taught how to deal with any trauma that we may have faced in our lifetimes. And so we do the easiest thing that society endorses, which is to ignore or numb the emotions that arise. Exploring our emotions is uncomfortable and takes time. But we can't escape from them, and so this chapter begins to look at ways to recognize, uncover, deal with and heal these emotions, which are an integral part of fertility.

How does trauma affect fertility?

Trauma influences our health and our propensity for disease, including our gynaecological health. Adverse events that lead to trauma, in particular those during childhood, have been shown to affect gynaecological conditions and fertility. For example, they can lead to chronic inflammation, oestrogen imbalance (more on this in Chapters 8 and 16) and may disrupt the immune system, all of which can directly contribute to infertility. Trauma alters our nervous system, so that a small or moderate amount of stress later on will induce a significant physiological response, setting the stage for disease. Women who have a history of childhood abuse have a risk of infertility that is more than 40 per cent higher than those without, and a more than 20 per cent higher risk of lower ovarian reserve or earlier menopause.

At the heart of trauma are emotions that weren't expressed openly, and so they express within the body, leaving biological traces. And trauma's roots therefore become entangled at the epigenetic, energetic, neurological and subconscious levels, activating a chronic degree of stress that keeps us in a permanent state of high alert and survival.

A stress response that is dysregulated – meaning a central nervous system that is highly sensitive, from being shaped by early life trauma – changes the chemical environment that impacts on the internal landscape of our bodies, contributing to conditions such as fibroids, polyps and dysfunctional uterine bleeding. Stress associated with trauma leads to inflammation of the central nervous system, or neuroinflammation, which can then lead to changes not only in cell signalling, but also epigenetic changes, nutrient deficiencies and changes in the gut microbiome. It can even lead to premature cell ageing, including that of your sperm and eggs.

The good news is that we can heal from trauma. We can bring subconscious emotions into conscious awareness, so that we have a chance to deal with them. We can learn to reshape our nervous system, changing our internal environment away from survival mode and towards connection and safety. We can connect our nervous system to joy and the authentic nature of who we are.

As with Annie, it may take the help of a counsellor, psychologist or therapist who can guide and support you through what may be a long process of healing, but it can also be one of the most crucial investments you make in yourself, including in your fertility.

There's a lot you can do yourself too. You can start to heal in small, everyday ways. The work that you'll do in the 12-week plan to calm your nervous system will contribute to the unpicking of trauma. This is one reason why stress is one of the pillars of TCP. The advice in the sex-and-relationships pillar (Chapter 10) is key here too: we can heal alongside others, in particular our partners.

Not only did healing her trauma help Annie to conceive, but it also meant there was less of a chance of it going on to affect her daughter. By doing that work, she will ultimately pass on the resilience and post-traumatic wisdom she built through her own healing.

The beginnings of your trauma

The majority of brain growth and organization takes place in the first few years of life, and so our childhood experiences shape our brain's internal architecture and how we experience our life.

Exposure to high levels of stress early in life can lead to epigenetic changes in our brain cells that direct how our bodies respond to adversity over our whole lifetime and our capacity to deal with stress, as well as how we perceive and respond to pain. These stressors might include physical, sexual or mental abuse, neglect and not having your emotional needs met; living with a parent with a mental illness or alcoholism; witnessing or experiencing domestic violence, poverty or racism. Or it may be that as a baby and growing up, your parents might not have been able to care for you in a way that made you feel safe. Or you may have been bullied or have lost a loved one, or other similarly distressing but common events.

In fact a baby's brain and nervous system can be shaped by trauma even before birth. A mother's stress can be transmitted in the womb through hormones and other chemicals. This prenatal period is crucial not just in terms of nutrients and other vital sustenance for the developing foetus, but also because it's when the baby's future mental, as well as physical, health is hardwired.

Studies done on animals have shown that stressful life experiences endured by either the mother while pregnant, or the child early in life, can end up affecting the receptors in the child's brain that respond to cortisol, the main stress hormone (this is one of the ways that the brain becomes hypersensitive to stress, or sensitized). In other words, the nervous system of the baby becomes epigenetically programmed by the mother, in what is emerging as a new field of science called neuroepigenetics. The child's stress axis is set in the womb, leading to changes in the brain and the whole nervous system. If you have been unhappy or stressed during your own pregnancy, please don't worry. It's impossible not to experience some level of emotional upset or turmoil in nine months. A baby has lots of capacity to change after birth too, especially with sensitive early mothering and attachment. What matters is being aware of it and doing something about it, which is what this book will help you with.

It's very likely that you inherited some form of trauma while you were in the womb, and you could pass it on to your future baby too, in the absence of healing. When we learn psychological resilience and how to deal with our stress in a healthy way, this is the legacy we give our children. As much as we can pass on an epigenome for stress, we can also pass on an epigenome for resilience. Our nervous systems are capable of incredible change and adaptation, through the process of neuroplasticity, meaning that we can learn to rewire and reshape our brain, by processing our emotions and learning how to self-regulate. Different experiences and environments will help to reorganize and restructure a dysregulated response.

How trauma can lead to, and impact upon, chronic gynaecological conditions

'It's all in your head', or 'There's not a lot more we can do', or 'We've tried all possible treatments' or 'We can't seem to find a cause.' How many times have you (or any other woman you know) been made to feel that you're making a fuss about a symptom, in particular one that's gynaecological? I have heard these stories from patients over and over again.

Being made to feel that your symptoms aren't real, or being invalidated in your experiences, is a form of gaslighting and it can often come from the medical establishment. It's a trauma in itself. It leaves women suffering because their symptoms often have to become serious before they are offered help. This leads them into a place of self-denial and suppression of their needs and emotions.

If you have given birth before, there is the trauma that can come from this. Modern-day obstetrics doesn't necessarily take into account how traumatic an emergency C-section, or interventions such as a ventouse (suction) delivery or even having stitches, can be, giving little follow-up to enable the patient to process what happened.

Historically, only 2 per cent of all medical research has been devoted to reproductive care. And when a woman goes to see the doctor, in far too many cases she has to push to get the necessary tests done and referrals made, at the risk of being labelled pushy or dramatic. And we wonder why it takes an average of eight years to diagnose endometriosis.

Stress and trauma can also lead to the symptoms of gynaecological conditions becoming worse. For example, an activated stress response can impact on the menstrual cycle, ovulation, fertility, libido and general well-being. As mentioned before, it also increases activity of the pain-processing regions of our brain, making chronic pain worse.

Let's use endometriosis as an example of how this can play out. Stress can accelerate the progression of endometriosis, generating more physical pain. If you do develop endometriosis, the dial in the central nervous system keeps getting turned up. Pain becomes amplified and the brain changes, not only in the regions responsible for processing pain, but also in those involved in processing emotions and memories. This abnormal signalling pattern will lead to more mental and emotional pain, which then promotes a bigger stress response. It's a vicious cycle.

Research has shown that changes in neurochemicals in response to stress affect the development of endometriosis. In fact experiencing significant trauma increases your risk of endometriosis by 80 per cent. Dr Holly Harris, who led a study into this, said, 'Both physical and sexual abuse were associated with endometriosis risk. And it's a strong association. There's also a dose response, meaning the risk increases with increasing severity and type of abuse.'

When a woman goes to seek help for her symptoms, perhaps at first her doctor doesn't recognize that she has endometriosis. She gets the message that the pain isn't real and is all in her head, generating even more trauma on top of that she may have experienced earlier in her life. She may then struggle to fall pregnant, and experience even more trauma in the form of comments and judgements about infertility that she internalizes, from other people, but also from the culture around her. And on it goes, a biological cascade of events in her body and brain, starting with trauma and leading to more pain and trauma, and often mental-health issues too. (There is more detail on the causes and treatments of endometriosis in Chapter 16.)

Why trauma affects us all – but some of us more than others

I've yet to meet a woman who hasn't suffered at least one form of abuse, denigration, subjugation, prejudice, humiliation or exploitation. In our patriarchal world, there isn't a woman who ends up escaping the effects of gender-biased adversities. Women do two-thirds of the world's work for one-tenth of the world's wages, and own less than one-hundredth of the world's estates.

This is not a book on trauma, and it is such a huge topic that there isn't room to go into all the ways in which it unfolds. But within infertility, there is also a significant amount of trauma coming from racial discrimination. A disproportionate number of women of colour don't have access to treatment. Black women's incidence of fibroids and Fallopian-tube diseases is higher, leaving them at a significant disadvantage when it comes to conceiving. Even when BMI, socio-economic status and the number of children is considered, African American women not only still have a higher incidence of fibroids, but tend to have larger tumours at diagnosis, an earlier age at diagnosis and more severe symptoms. Black women also have a twofold risk of hysterectomy compared to Caucasian women, and a sevenfold risk of myomectomy (the surgical removal of fibroids).

For some, the trauma may not be as deeply rooted as this. But even small consistent put-downs can eventually amount to trauma. Any situations that made you feel insecure, anxious, emotionally suppressed, neglected or in conflict may have led your brain to be rewired, to become sensitive to stress in order to prioritize survival. And as we'll see in Part 3, this has consequences when it comes to gynaecological conditions.

How we relate to the world around us, and to the social experiences we have, is an inseparable part of our well-being. Trauma can look like any of the following:

* **Issues relating to belonging**, such as compromising ourselves and our feelings in order to show we belong.

* **Issues around relationships**, such as dealing with abuse, abandonment, exploitation, betrayal or co-dependency.

* **Issues around self-esteem** (our sense of integrity and authenticity).

All of these can set in motion a series of biological events that can damage our health and lead to disease.

For example, one possible effect of trauma is early puberty in girls (defined as puberty before the age of eight), which is becoming more common. And this sets off various mechanisms that lead to premature ageing, diseases and infertility. Early puberty also brings a double whammy of trauma: it hypersexualizes girls, who may then experience further trauma through assault, or anxieties generated by unwanted attention or precocious expectations.

But our collective consciousness is changing. Women all over the world are standing up to express the wounds of their past, in order to heal themselves and future generations. It's happening in the MeToo movement exposing sexual violence and exploitation, as well as the Black Lives Matter movement, where generational racism is finally being challenged. More recently, we see it in the launch of the Women's Health Strategy for England. After thousands of women shared their traumatizing medical experiences, the government announced a new action plan for healthcare, focused on filling the gaps in treatment and righting inequalities.

Women's voices are finally being listened to, in the UK and hopefully further afield. I believe this is the first step towards providing the courage so many of us need in order to listen to our inner guidance, return to our intuition and start trusting our own bodies and the wisdom they hold. No matter what has happened to us, we have the potential to transform, spiritually, emotionally and physically. Trauma can become the catalyst for unfathomable growth and a capacity for love and healing.

A special kind of trauma: the Mother Wound

This is a specific type of trauma that I see coming up a lot in patients, probably because the first call to heal it often comes via infertility. The process of wanting to become a mother may deeply remind us of our relationship with our own mothers – our first bond and our greatest teacher in how we love and seek safety in the world.

This is the relationship upon which all others are based. Whereas it can be a source of great empowerment, it can also be a place of shame, anger and resentment. Chances are that, no matter how loving and nurturing your mother is or may have been, there will be aspects of the relationship that caused pain for you both. In the present, this can play out as difficult dynamics between you and your mother.

The roots of the Mother Wound go way deeper than the relationship that we have with our mother, according to one of the experts on this, the therapist Bethany Webster. She says it's a set of dysfunctional coping mechanisms, including the sacrifice of full potential and the denial of our authentic needs, that can jeopardize our relationships, including the one we have with ourselves. It originates from a pattern of internalized values that places limitations on women. It's based on the patriarchal lie that there is something inherently wrong, less valued or damaged about a woman or a daughter.

Our mothers absorbed and lived this. And then, as children, our need to survive and gain approval from our mother meant that we adopted their unconscious patterns and programmes of behaviour. All of us carry this wound, to a lesser or greater extent. Even if we choose not to make the same sacrifices as previous generations, we fear rejection for making that choice, and so we are left with shame and difficulty in our relationship with our mother.

CASE STUDY

Meera, who'd been trying to conceive for three years and was now in her early thirties, had PCOS, irregular periods, PMS and a complicated and fractured relationship with her mother. As a child, she felt that her mother was either emotionally unavailable or overbearing. She felt that whatever she did wasn't good enough, that the decisions she was making in her life were wrong, and questioned whether she would ever be a good mother. Meera's unhealthy eating habits had started early in life, driven by her dysregulated emotions.

She revealed that she'd struggled with her weight for most of her life, and it became evident this had a strong emotional connection for her, being her way of trying to diminish herself and her own needs as a woman. Her PCOS had started in her teens; I told her that PCOS can sometimes carry the emotional residue of a woman pressured into masculinizing herself to survive in a world where women are traditionally seen as the lesser sex. Pushing herself at work was a way to try and gain her mother's approval.

She'd been on the pill for fifteen years, which kept her PMS under control. But it also robbed her of a chance to engage with the hidden trauma. Now that she was struggling to conceive, all her old insecurities and unresolved grief from the relationship with her mother were beginning to surface. She and her partner couldn't afford to have IVF, and her BMI precluded them from having government funding.

As soon as they came to see me, I started the couple on TCP, beginning with Meera's eating habits and lack of exercise. I suggested she get some emotional support too. With the help of a shaman and reiki practitioner to deal with painful emotions as they arose, and with the support of techniques in emotional self-regulation, such as mindfulness and meditation, Meera started addressing the deep-seated issues concerning her relationship with her mother.

It was an intensely emotional process. As she did the work, she said that her intimate relationship with her partner began to improve too. I asked her to write a letter to her mother, to express everything she wanted to say and never could. In doing this, Meera recognized her mum as a human with her own wounds, and she was also finally able to tell her when and how she had felt let down. I encouraged her to perform a little ceremony of burning the letter, which Meera said gave her an immediate sense of relief.

I also encouraged her to start mothering and nurturing herself in the way she wished she'd received from her mother, looking after her needs in small steps. Within a few weeks Meera had lost weight. For the first time that she could remember, her periods became regular. As her relationship with her body healed, the one with her mother did too.

A few weeks later, Meera found out she was naturally pregnant for the first time. She went on to have a beautiful and healthy baby boy.

You might recognize the Mother Wound in you, from any of these patterns of behaviour:

* Resentment towards your mother (or your children)

* A need to conform to a certain view of womanhood

* Putting others' needs above your own

* You were – or are – a 'good girl'

* You are a people-pleaser

❋ You hesitate to express the truth of who you are, in case it's judged or disapproved of

❋ Difficulty in coping with failure

❋ You are fearful of overshadowing others with your own success

❋ You over-extend yourself or sacrifice your own needs for the sake of others

❋ You never feel that you're enough

❋ You act small, so as not to threaten others

❋ You rarely or never prioritize taking care of yourself.

This pattern is handed down, from mother to mother. If any of this sounds like you, chances are your mother may have passed this on to you, because it's what she inherited.

One area of fertility that gives a window into the Mother Wound consists of problems with the womb and pattern of menstruation (more on this in Chapter 15), as well as problems with the menstrual cycle such as heavy menstrual bleeding and PMS (see the box on page 71). By the way, there is a Father Wound too; and men can be affected by the Mother Wound, as you'll see in Chapter 11.

Pregnancy is another trigger for the Mother Wound. Women describe how being pregnant or becoming a mother brought them closer to their mothers, but also deepened the trauma of any abuse, neglect, abandonment, control or subjugation. Many of these emotional issues can manifest as physical symptoms in pregnancy, when a woman hasn't had an opportunity to recognize and address aspects of this wounding beforehand. Dr Oscar Serrallach, a post-natal specialist, outlines how the Mother Wound can also come from post-natal depletion, when new mothers who lack support feel isolated while struggling to fulfil all the physical and emotional demands of a baby. If a mother hasn't got the physical energy or mental clarity to look after herself and her child, she can hardly be expected to be the mother she would want to be.

If you can deal with the Mother Wound before becoming pregnant, then you won't risk passing it down to your child. In fact simply by recognizing these generational patterns that have embedded themselves in our cellular tissue, we can develop new habits that change these patterns and programming.

How trauma is inherited

We've seen the power of the epigenome in influencing our health and our ability to get pregnant; trauma is yet another piece of that epigenetic puzzle. There is now an overwhelming amount of evidence that trauma can be transmitted epigenetically through at least three generations, as seen through studies on famines. For example, the children of Holocaust survivors had trauma-induced epigenetic modification of a particular gene, even when they grew up hearing nothing about the events of the time.

These biological scars are passed on to future generations, unless trauma is processed into something positive. How you deal with your trauma will not only impact on your fertility, but can also shape your future baby's nervous system, and their entire blueprint for health. This makes it a crucial part of preconception care. And with the right post-natal support, even what happened in the womb can be reversed through bonding and attachment with the child.

Mother Wound trauma has its own kind of biological inheritance too. There's a type of DNA that's inherited only from mother to mother – mitochondrial DNA. The mitochondria are the energy-producing batteries of our cells, part of the internal environment of the cell that regulates, fine-tunes and manages cell behaviour. Like the cell membrane, the mitochondria play a role in deciding which external epigenetic factors reach the DNA of the cell. Among their other important roles, they are also responsible for releasing significant hormones in the placenta during pregnancy, as well as for producing many of our sex hormones. And so, via your mitochondrial DNA, you can trace generations of women – your mother's mother, and so on – in the tissue that you're made up of.

Our maternal lineage is a blessing, even if the relationship with your mother was fractured and complicated, as many are. But being in denial of this wound and/or becoming your mother's opposite will rob you of the chance to carve out your own identity as a mother, because you'll be resisting and focusing on what you don't want. Like a baby stuck in the birth canal, you have to live through the painful contractions of healing and clearing up the emotional bonds of the past that hold you back.

Having therapy may be the right way to heal. There's no shame in this; it's one of the most empowering things you can do. But you can do a lot for yourself too. The five pillars for conception, which come next in the book, plus the 12-week plan (see page 198) will support you on this journey of reconnecting with yourself, using journaling prompts. Like Meera, you'll also be guided through the process of writing a letter to your mother (which you won't send).

Just as trauma has the capacity to set up destructive cascades within our bodies, so we also have the chance to override this by understanding that we can use trauma to heal and bring greater awareness to our bodies, nurturing and healing, as well as growing into the fullness of who we were always destined to be.

WHAT IS YOUR PMS TRYING TO TELL YOU?

In situations where our hormonal, immune and nervous systems are activated, such as in the lead-up to menstruation, our old memories and unexpressed emotions can be brought to the forefront. And so the anger, rage, volatility and sadness you may feel during PMS may actually be symptoms of previous traumas finally getting a chance to express themselves through your body. As little girls, we may have been told our emotions weren't appropriate — part of the Mother Wound — and so we're made to feel bad and that there's something wrong with us, leading us to suppress and deny our emotions. The medical profession also encourages this view in the way we treat PMS, which is essentially to cover it up. Being on the pill, which suppresses our own hormones, has left us divorced from our feelings, instead of looking at what they're trying to show us. But the window before menstruation is in fact one of the greatest insights into our emotions and our trauma and the parts of ourselves that need attention and healing. In the 12-week plan you'll journal your thoughts and feelings that come up – a basis to start exploring the source of some of these emotions, to help you to heal and to improve your symptoms.

Techniques you'll use to look at deep emotions

These are two of the tools you'll be using during the 12-week plan to help bring up emotions so that you can process them.

Breathwork

Breathing techniques tap into your body and nervous system, setting off a positive neurological, endocrine and immune cascade of messengers that lead to a reduction in stress hormones, a shift towards the parasympathetic nervous system and improving a measure of stress called heart-rate variability (see page 119). In the 12-week plan you can practise this daily, or as needed. Breathing also helps to improve the amount of oxygen that our cells are getting. Research has shown that after following eight weeks of diaphragmatic breathing sessions, participants had lower levels of the major stress hormone, cortisol.

Therapies for trauma

These techniques can be done with the support of a therapist.

❋   **Emotional Freedom Technique (EFT)**: this is a method you can learn from an expert to help release trauma; it involves tapping into acupoints across the body while recognizing negative feelings, and then turning them into positive affirmations and statements of self-acceptance. It has been shown to help even those with severe levels of trauma, such as survivors of abuse and post-war veterans, with MRI scans confirming positive brain changes as a result.

* **Eye Movement Desensitization and Reprocessing (EMDR):** this involves left- and right-eye movements that are therapist-directed, helping to access the parasympathetic nervous system — something our ancient ancestors were used to doing; if it is done while recalling adverse experiences, it reinforces a link between the experience and a sense of peace and calm. This has become an evidence-based treatment for PTSD in war veterans.

* **Tension and Trauma-Release Exercises (TRE):** this is a simple set of exercises that help the body to release stress, tension and trauma. It was developed by Dr David Berceli, who observed communities traumatized by war. He discovered that by inducing the body's natural tremor-mechanisms to release trauma, there was a big reduction in the need for both psychotherapy and medication. They are exercises that can be done to trigger a natural tremor reflex, and may be found online and on YouTube.

PART 2
The Conception Plan Pillars

CHAPTER 6

Pillar 1: Nutrition

Food provides the raw materials for producing healthy sperm and eggs. It's also the key to creating a fertile inner environment. What you eat has a huge impact on how your genes express themselves, so nutrition is one of the main ways in which we get to influence our epigenome. For you to be fertile and for a baby to thrive, you need real, nourishing food.

There are even more reasons for being committed to a positive way of eating. It will not only reduce the chance of infertility, but will ultimately influence your long-term health. During pregnancy the placenta draws on your stores of vitamins and minerals. And so how you eat now will affect not only the post-natal period, but also future pregnancies, the menopause and beyond. And your baby's life too; research shows that the food babies are exposed to while in the womb affects their food choices later in life. Modern, processed foods are often not fertile-friendly. They tend to be high in sugar and vegetable oils, which negatively interfere with hormonal signals between different organs, including the uterus, the placenta and the ovaries. Eating these foods in pregnancy can lead to an increase in the risk of diabetes and pre-eclampsia (a condition that involves raised blood pressure in pregnancy, with wider consequences), and can also negatively influence the growth and development of the baby.

The foods we eat can also encourage the production of new nerve cells within us and within babies *in utero*, increasing the number of neural circuits and therefore something called 'synaptic plasticity', which helps to build greater resilience to stress as well as improving overall mental health.

Eating to conceive

This chapter will help you become conscious of the effect of food on your body. TCP eating isn't about prescriptive rules, nor does it condone any severe form of dieting or a particular diet. It aims to do three things: 1) maximize the intake of the nutrients you need for fertility, your health and the future health of your baby; 2) maximize their absorption; and 3) minimize any unwanted foods, additives or chemicals.

Please don't feel judged, or stressed about being perfect, when it comes to food. Focusing on what you eat can be emotionally tricky, especially if you've struggled in your relationship with food. But if you've only previously thought of food as calories or fat, this is a great time to start seeing it as a source of health and nourishment.

Follow TCP guidance *most* of the time and you'll notice that your tastes and cravings change, so that you naturally start to make better and healthier decisions. In fact, looking after yourself in this way can help deepen your connection with your intuition, so that your choices become guided by your body's needs. You'll also feel more replenished, positive, focused, rejuvenated and energetic. It's never too late to start!

TCP nutrition-pillar guidelines: simple steps to take now

The key to healthy eating is to incorporate foods that send the right messages to your cells, encouraging behaviour that promotes well-being and fertility, and eliminating or reducing those foods that do the opposite. Let's now have a look to see what foods we need to eat more of and those we need to avoid, in order to create the optimal conditions for health and conception.

Do your shopping mindfully

To increase crop yields, most food is grown with herbicides and pesticides. And most soil is depleted in minerals, which means that our food is too. Then there are genetically modified (GM) foods, which are becoming increasingly common; and some animals that we eat are fed GMO grains, so we can end up ingesting them via the food chain.

We still need detailed studies to understand the effect of GM foods on humans, but animal studies suggest there are effects on both the animal that eats it and its offspring, including effects on fertility.

Try to buy local, organic and/or at farmers' markets to help you cut down on GM, pesticides, insecticides and fungicides. Some foods don't necessarily need to be organic, such as: bananas, avocados, aubergines, kiwis, onions, pineapples, watermelons, sweet potatoes, mangoes and cabbages. However, there are others where organic really is best, including: strawberries, peaches, blueberries, apples, grapes, soy, spinach, squash, celery, lettuce, kale and chard.

However, if there's one thing you buy organic, make it meat. Organic animal products contain a higher concentration of nutrients and fewer hormones, antibiotics, pesticides and herbicides.

Build a fertile microbiome

You've probably heard about the gut microbiome: the billions of microbes that help digest our food. Did you know that they also help with the absorption of some nutrients and make others, are involved in eliminating toxins, look after the health of our mitochondria and act as our immune system's first line of defence? To do all those jobs well, you need a wide variety of microbes – a diverse microbiome – with a good balance of beneficial bacteria keeping the harmful ones in check.

The microbiome also plays several roles in fertility. Some microbes make up what's called the oestrobolome, as they are responsible for oestrogen metabolism in both men and women. Also, a lack of diversity in the gut microbiome has been linked with some gynaecological conditions, as well as problems in conceiving. It can influence, for example, the development of PCOS, endometriosis, obesity and endometrial hyperplasia (thickening of the womb lining, leading to heavy periods and potentially cancer).

We have microbiomes not only in the gut, but elsewhere in and on the body, including in the vagina and on/in the testes. New research is showing that imbalances in those microbiomes may also be related to infertility.

Some studies show that having a balanced gut microbiome can reduce our response to stress. The gut is often referred to as the 'second brain' and for good reason, as this is where many neurotransmitters – including 90 per cent of the feel-good hormone serotonin – are produced, as well as other chemicals that influence mood. And remember that the central nervous system, including the brain, is one of the most important regulators of fertility. It's also part of the epigenome – that means that changes in our bacteria can lead to genetic changes.

The problem is that the modern (over-) use of antibiotics, anti-microbials and pasteurization wipes out all bacteria, both good and bad. Of course you don't want potentially harmful pathogens. But a microbiome that's out of balance enables harmful microbes to thrive, leading to inflammation – the body's natural response to foreign invaders or injury. And when inflammation becomes chronic, it can lead to disease, including infertility and endometriosis.

Everything you eat feeds the bacteria in your gut. Eating junk food regularly will encourage more pathological strains of bacteria to thrive. However, eating vegetables (and lots of them) feeds the bacteria that you want.

So follow these veggie rules: rainbow, raw, steamed, seasonal and fermented:

* **Rainbow**: fresh fruit and vegetables in season contain lots of antioxidant phytonutrients, which protect our tissues from stress and damage. The more intense the colour, the more phytonutrients a vegetable or fruit contains. Eating colourful rainbow foods can lead to what is referred to as xenohormesis. This involves certain phytonutrients having epigenetic effects to upregulate the gene expression of detoxification enzymes, and it includes nutrients from turmeric, resveratrol from berries, allicin from garlic, quercetin from fruit and vegetables, and green tea.

* **Red fruit and vegetables** contain lycopene, which is important for prostate health and has been shown to help improve sperm counts. It is found in tomatoes, watermelon and red peppers.

* **Green cruciferous vegetables**, such as Brussels sprouts, broccoli, cabbage, kale and turnips, contain a phytonutrient called diindolylmethane (DIM), which is important in helping the body to metabolize oestrogen. DIM also helps if oestrogen levels are too high, which is related to infertility as well as conditions such as PCOS, endometriosis and fibroids. In men, DIM helps to improve testosterone levels.

* **Purple fruit and veg**, such as blueberries, aubergines, red cabbage, plums, grapes and red onions, are rich in anthocyanins, which have anti-inflammatory and antioxidant properties.

* **Beige vegetables**, such as garlic and onions, have important antibacterial properties, and are prebiotics, which means they feed the gut microbiome.

* **Some raw, some steamed**: veg are best eaten fresh and either raw or lightly cooked, because antioxidant levels reduce with longer periods of storage and with heating. Gentle cooking, such as steaming, releases the vitamins and minerals from the cell walls. And blending raw fruit and vegetables in the form of a smoothie breaks down the fibre, enabling you to absorb their nutrients more easily.

* **Seasonal**: food that's in season often tastes better, is fresher and more nutritious, because it hasn't had to travel far and therefore hasn't had to be treated with various chemicals to help preserve it. It has also not required as much packaging or processing, meaning it's better for the planet too. Not to mention that seasonal food harnesses nature's innate wisdom concerning what our bodies need most at that particular time, providing hydrating fruit and vegetables in summer, and vegetables such as artichokes and asparagus in spring to help with natural detoxification.

* **Fermented**: food that's been activated by fermentation or sprouting is abundant in raw enzymes and probiotics, which

allows for better food absorption. Sprouting involves soaking nuts, seeds and grains until they sprout, releasing their full nutritional value, because the processes encourage plants to activate enzymes that liberate bound-up nutrients and create new ones by converting stored starch and fatty acids into proteins and vitamins that are bioavailable, or able to be absorbed and used effectively by the body. Fermented and sprouted vegetables are also easier to digest, because they have had undesirable enzyme inhibitors, among other irritants, deactivated. Buying vegetables in this form, and incorporating sauerkraut, kimchi and pickles into your diet, comes with nutritional benefits and is great for supporting the microbiome.

Reduce sugar

A high sugar intake can lead to lower fertility in several ways, as you'll see below. But one major way is glycation. This is a process where high sugar levels lead to advanced glycation end products (AGEs), where tissues harden and become stiff, just as bread becomes when it's toasted.

You might have heard of AGEs in terms of their ageing effects on skin, but there are also receptors for AGEs in the uterus and ovaries. If there's an accumulation of AGEs in the uterus, it can become inflamed and affect implantation of the embryo. Women with PCOS have been found to have high levels of AGEs and, when these accumulate at the ovarian follicles, they can give rise to premature ovarian ageing. In men, the quality of DNA found in sperm is linked with high levels of AGEs.

Not only do you want to avoid making AGEs, but you want to avoid eating them too. They are found in any food that has turned brown during cooking.

To reduce AGEs in your food and your body:

* Avoid processed and especially sugary foods.

* Avoid barbecued, toasted, grilled and fried foods – these contain AGEs.

* Increase slow cooking, poaching, steaming and casseroling. This avoids the brown layer on foods that contain AGEs.

* Use marinades that are acidic, such as lemon and vinegar, to help reduce the formation of AGEs.

It's fine to eat some healthy sugars in fruit. And much smaller amounts of unprocessed sugar, such as coconut to replace white and brown sugar. But avoid high-sugar foods, including fizzy drinks, jam, sweets, cakes, biscuits, energy bars and drinks.

Check the labels. Lots of foods are packed with hidden sugars, in particular in low-fat versions of processed foods and sauces. On the label, look out for and avoid corn syrup, fructose, sucrose, malt, barley syrup, maltose, dextrose, beet juice, maple syrup, brown rice syrup and corn sweeteners. Avoid glucose-fructose syrup in particular, which is found in some jams, ice cream and biscuits.

Focus on good fats

Eating the right sorts of fat is key, not least because they contain fatty acids that help to make hormones, support ovulation and create sperm. Fatty acids are also an integral and crucial part of cell membranes. And as explained in Chapter 1, cell membranes are not just barriers, but actively regulate how well you absorb nutrients, as well as how cells communicate with each other and with their DNA-containing cell nucleus.

Eating good fats also supports the microbiome and the immune system, and helps to facilitate blood clotting and the absorption of vitamins. Good fats also reduce inflammation and help keep blood sugar balanced. The wrong kinds of fats can have a negative impact: they drive inflammation, inhibit ovulation and interfere with hormone signalling.

These are the fats to eat more and less of:

* **Eat more:** unsaturated fats. These contain both Omega 3 and Omega 6, and you need the right balance of these, in favour of Omega 3. We tend to get more Omega 6 fats in our diets, so focus on Omega 3 instead. Up to 95 per

cent of the population is estimated to have low Omega 3 levels. Omega 3 is important for supporting ovulation, building cell membranes and sperm, improving the chances of implantation and enhancing blood flow to the uterus and placenta. These are the best fats to help the central nervous system to function optimally too. Omega 3 has been shown to help reduce the incidence of endometriosis and to increase pregnancy and live birth rates with IVF, with a 1 per cent increase in consumption linked to an 8 per cent increase in success at pregnancy; and to reduce FSH, which can often be high in women with lower ovarian reserve, helping to improve the chances of conception. And when it comes to men, Omega 3 is important in sperm function, integrity and number.

Sources: raw, cold-pressed plant, seed and nut oils, including olive oil, flaxseed, sesame seed, chia and hemp-seed oil. Avocados. Fish such as salmon, herring and sardines, cod-liver oil and fish oils. Eggs (these also contain cholesterol, which is important in building hormones). Try to go for grass-fed dairy and organic eggs as these contain more Omega 3.

✳ **Eat some:** saturated fats. These used to have a bad reputation, but recently they have been recognized for their value, in small doses, helping to increase the bioavailability and absorption of some vitamins and minerals. They provide cholesterol, which is essential for the synthesis of hormones and cell membranes.

Sources: grass-fed organic meat and poultry, coconut oil, ghee.

✳ **Avoid:** processed or refined vegetable oils. Most of the fats in the modern diet come from refined vegetable oils, because they are cheap. They can change structure – oxidize – in the bottle and when heating, which produces toxic compounds and free radicals (unstable atoms that can damage cells, causing illness and ageing). Refined fats contribute to processes that can lead to infertility and miscarriage, as well as female and male reproductive-health conditions.

Sources: refined cooking oils such as vegetable, corn, sunflower, safflower, soybean, rapeseed (canola, not cold-pressed) and margarine.

❊ It's fine to eat minimally-processed vegetable oils cold in salad dressings, but look for cold-pressed oils in dark glass bottles. For heating or cooking, use butter, coconut oil, grass-fed ghee and olive oil.

❊ **Avoid:** trans fats. These are a known health risk, increasing the likelihood of heart disease, stroke and Alzheimer's, among other conditions. But they have also been linked to infertility, problems with ovulation and endometriosis. They are made when heat and pressure are used to change vegetable oil to a semi-solid product, which increases shelf life. On food labels they may be called partially hydrogenated oils, or mono- and diglycerides. UK manufacturers have promised to reduce them, but they are still in some processed foods and fast foods, including baked goods, margarine and ice cream.

Enjoy the right carbs

'Carbohydrates' is the term for all sugars, starches and fibres. We need good carbs to build a favourable microbiome, regulate inflammation and support our immunity. Good carbs have a low Glycaemic Index (GI), which means that they raise our blood sugar slowly. Another measure of this is the Glycaemic Load (GL), which is how much a portion of a food raises your blood sugar.

You want to avoid carbs with a high GI and GL. These include sugars, but also white rice, white pasta, potatoes (not boiled and cooled potatoes), fries and low-fibre breakfast cereals. High-GI carbs raise blood sugar fast. This leads to an increase in insulin to clear up all the sugar. Then your blood-sugar levels go down and you experience the typical post-carb slump and sleepiness. The adrenal glands try to compensate by secreting more of the stress hormone, cortisol. This promotes inflammation and when you're making cortisol, you're not making sex hormones. Eating high-GL carbs is associated with ovulatory infertility, whereas eating wholegrain carbs with a low GI has been shown to improve implantation and live births by up to 20 per cent in patients undergoing IVF.

The carbs you want to eat are low-GI carbs. These are made from multiple sugar molecules linked together, which take the body longer to digest and therefore don't lead to sugar and insulin swings. As a rule, go for less processed, more wholegrain carbs and root vegetables. Wholegrains have more nutritional value because they include the nutrient-rich outer shell, with more fibre, antioxidants and phytonutrients. Sources of low-GI carbs are quinoa, spelt, bulgur wheat and brown rice, as well as parsnips, sweet potatoes, beetroot, carrots and other roots.

We do need carbs for compounds called glyconutrients, which help communication between cells. Sources include aloe vera, mushrooms and a range of fruit and vegetables, including avocados, strawberries, cabbage, chestnuts, pineapples, bananas, cranberries, tomatoes, blackberries and spinach.

Eat plenty of quality protein, particularly from plants

Proteins support the function of every cell in our bodies. They're necessary to build our tissues and hormones, as well as for egg development and sperm maturation.

Meat and fish are good sources. There is concern about environmental pollutants carried by fish, but the benefits of eating seafood appear to significantly outweigh the potential adverse effects. Couples who consume two servings of seafood a week had a 60 per cent shorter time to pregnancy, and more than a 10 per cent lowered risk of infertility. Eating fish is associated with improved progesterone levels, a positive effect on early embryo development and an increase in libido, especially when seafood was eaten by the couple on the same day.

However, avoid bigger fish, such as tuna and swordfish, as they contain mercury. Eat wild rather than farmed fish. And eat shellfish cooked, not raw, when you're trying to conceive. Good fish to eat are salmon, sardines, cod, sea bass and herring.

However, plant protein is the key. Studies have shown that deriving most of your protein from plants can lead to an improvement of ovulatory infertility by as much as 50 per cent. So include combinations of these: buckwheat, brown rice, lentils, chickpeas, mung beans, quinoa, nut butters and seeds.

There are some proteins you definitely want to avoid. Processed meats contain artificial preservatives, including MSG, nitrates and nitrites, which have been correlated with inflammation, nerve damage and diabetes. Also, when you are pregnant, avoid raw meat, as well as game meat, liver products and pâtés, as they may carry a small risk of toxoplasmosis, which can cause miscarriage.

Be discerning about dairy

Opt for full-fat grass-fed dairy food that has a better balance of fats; it's associated with a lower risk of infertility due to problems with ovulation, reducing this risk by up to 66 per cent, whereas low-fat dairy has the opposite effect. If you drink plant milks such as almond, cashew and coconut, go for one without added sugar or chemicals, but fortified with calcium, iodine and other vitamins. Plant-based milks do not contain the same vitamins and minerals and have a reduced protein content compared to dairy.

Embrace fermented foods

A regular intake of probiotics – live microorganisms – will allow the good bacteria in our guts to proliferate. This includes fermented foods, such as kefir, yoghurt, kombucha, sauerkraut and pickled vegetables; fibre-rich foods, such as vegetables and wholegrains, apples, flaxseeds, chia seeds; and healthy oils and fats.

Choose better-made bread

Aim for high-nutrition, high-fibre bread, ideally organic, to minimize the pesticide residue and additives that are found in a lot of mass-produced bread. The best option is sprouted grain bread, but it's hard to come by, and the next best is sourdough. Sourdough bread provides prebiotics for the gut microbiome, and because it's made through a longer fermentation process, it's easier to digest, also improving bioavailability of the fibre that it contains, as well as having a lower glycaemic index.

Be careful about soya-based products

Soya-based products contain goitrogens, which can disrupt thyroid function; and also phytoestrogens, which can interfere with hormone signalling. Traditional tofu, miso and other soy products are very nutritious, as they undergo a process of soaking and fermentation to neutralize the harmful substances and promote microbial growth. However, the commercially made soy products now in supermarkets, including soya milk and tofu, have little nutritional value and contain the compounds listed above, which when consumed in larger or more frequent quantities may have detrimental effects on reproductive function. Organic fermented soy products such as tamari and miso are fine in moderation.

Limit your caffeine

Caffeine can increase stress in the body, reduce blood flow to the reproductive organs and negatively impact on implantation. Up to one cup of coffee, two of black tea or three of green tea per day is okay. A 2017 study showed that consuming more than one daily cup of coffee (or its caffeine equivalent) increased the risk of early miscarriage. And having more than two cups a day more than doubled this risk. The risk of miscarriage also applies to men who consume too much caffeine, as their sperm are affected.

Drinking tea may be better: it contains hypoxanthine, which helps to support egg maturation, and antioxidant polyphenols. Green tea has far more of the latter than black tea. Make sure you also count the caffeine in chocolate and other caffeinated drinks in your daily amount.

Finally, yes, it might be time to give up drinking . . .

Giving up drinking alcohol for what might turn out to be a long preconception period may feel tough and may be unrealistic for some. However, during the preconception period you and your partner should go alcohol-free as much as possible.

If you're having fertility treatment, it's been shown that alcohol consumption – both male and female – can impact on the success rate. There may be times when you feel like resorting to alcohol (such as if an IVF round isn't successful), but try to keep it to a minimum and go back to abstinence when you can. If drinking is your way of releasing stress, try to find other ways to do so (see the 12-week plan).

Alcohol damages fertility in multiple ways. In men, it's toxic to sperm, reducing its quality and motility and increasing abnormalities. It reduces testosterone as well as libido, and increases the incidence of erectile dysfunction. In women, alcohol can reduce ovulation, create hormone imbalances and increase the chance of miscarriage. In both sexes, it affects the ability of the body to absorb nutrients from food and can interfere with the action of folate. However, if you or your partner find yourselves reaching for a small amount sporadically, make it red wine as this contains resveratrol, which is an antioxidant.

Remember that foetal abnormalities can start even before you know you're pregnant, including development issues with the heart and the central nervous system. Drinking also increases the chances of preterm birth and low birth weight. Cutting out alcohol completely is advised if you're pregnant, but also if your period is late.

Key fertile vitamins and minerals

Vitamin A

Vitamin A is important for the follicle and endometrium, as well as for progesterone production and to help protect sperm from oxidative stress. In the foetus it's needed for the normal development of the foetal heart, eyes, ears, bones and limbs and helps to oversee the action of growth hormone. In pregnancy, synthetic vitamin A – retinol – isn't recommended because an accumulation in the body can lead to birth defects. The plant-based carotenoid type of vitamin A is fine, as it's water-soluble, so it does not accumulate. Beta-carotene helps to sustain the earlier stages of a pregnancy.

Sources: yellow squash, red and yellow peppers, tomatoes, carrots, melon and sweet potatoes. Carotenoids become more bioavailable to the body when the vegetables are gently cooked or blended in a smoothie or soup.

B vitamins

You've doubtless heard of folate being key to foetal health, but other B vitamins are also key in fertility. Getting adequate amounts can help reduce the risk of failed IVF and miscarriage. They counter oxidative stress, which can help to protect eggs and sperm. They're also vital in helping the liver to metabolize excess hormones, as well as in blood-sugar regulation. In women, they're important in ovulation and implantation. Optimal levels of B vitamins in follicular fluid – the fluid surrounding the egg cells – have been linked to better fertility outcomes. In men, they affect sperm DNA, quality and count. Getting adequate amounts can also help to reduce levels of homocysteine, an amino acid that can reduce male and female fertility as well as increase the chance of miscarriage.

In the foetus, B vitamins help to build the nervous system, muscles and bones. They're essential in reducing the risk of neural-tube defects and chromosomal abnormalities. The reason folate is such a crucial micronutrient is that it oversees the process of methylation in cells. This is one of the main ways in which gene expression is controlled, as well as keeping DNA stable. Most people (50 per cent of the general population, but thought to be as high as 70 per cent in Caucasians) carry a gene mutation called MTHFR, so they are unable to metabolize the usual kind of folic acid; check that your supplement contains the natural version of folate, methyl tetrahydrofolate, which bypasses this gene. In fact if you have this mutation, taking folic acid can actually deplete your natural stores of folate, as it can impact on the MTHFR gene to lead to even slower metabolization. If you have diabetes or inflammatory bowel disorder, or if you or your child have had neural-tube defects and/or are overweight, then you need higher doses of folate.

Sources: lentils, beans, potatoes. You can add nutritional yeast to meals.

Vitamin C

This vitamin is one of the main antioxidants the body needs in order to combat free radicals, which are unstable atoms that are often caused by inflammation, which can cause disease and ageing. It's key in the corpus luteum (a normal cyst that develops on an ovary during the luteal phase of each cycle following ovulation, which plays a vital role in fertility and early pregnancy), encouraging the production of progesterone. In men, vitamin C can help to preserve DNA integrity.

Sources: citrus fruit, kiwis, strawberries, cherries, tomatoes and green vegetables such as kale, peas, asparagus and broccoli.

Vitamin D

This vitamin acts more like a hormone rather than a micronutrient; there are vitamin D receptors on the ovaries, the endometrium and the placenta, as well as in sperm and the testicles. It supports ovulation as well as being an antioxidant. It's also important for pregnancy, because adequate prenatal vitamin D has been shown to help protect against gestational diabetes and pre-eclampsia, as well as health problems in children, such as allergies and asthma.

Sources: we get most of our vitamin D from sun exposure. Go in the sun for twenty minutes a day during off-peak hours (before 11 a.m., after 3 p.m.) with bare arms and legs. However, most of us need a supplement year-round, and especially in winter. Food sources are cod-liver oil, egg yolks and mushrooms.

Vitamin E

This is another important antioxidant that helps to protect cell membranes from free-radical damage, as well as protecting sperm and improving its ability to fertilize an egg. It also acts as a natural anti-coagulant (preventing blood-clot formation), which can help to reduce the risk of miscarriage and promote implantation.

Sources: (cold-pressed) oils, nuts, seeds; beet and spinach greens; red peppers, broccoli, avocados, eggs, wholegrains.

Vitamin K

Vitamin K is important for blood clotting, helping to prevent excessive bruising and bleeding, and is also necessary for efficient vitamin D absorption. It can benefit those with PCOS and endometriosis, as well as low sperm counts.

Sources: eating green vegetables, such as kale and cabbage, helps the bacteria in the gut to produce vitamin K, making the microbiome key. Vitamin K is also found in grass-fed ghee.

Iron

Iron is needed to help build the blood supply, which is especially important as blood circulation increases significantly during pregnancy. Iron deficiency is common in women, particularly after pregnancy and pregnancy loss, and if you have heavy periods. Strengthening your microbiome will help with the absorption of iron, as will eating a source of vitamin C with every meal, soaking legumes and grains before cooking, and avoiding tea, coffee and wine with meals.

Sources: meat and leafy green vegetables; dried fruit, nuts, legumes and grains.

Zinc

Zinc is important for hormone balance. In women, it has a role in ovulation; and in men, in making sperm and improving their motility.

Sources: wholegrains, nuts, seeds, beans, oysters and red meat.

Iodine

This is a key factor in thyroid function, which affects fertility. In men, thyroid hormones affect reproduction by altering testosterone levels, and low levels of iodine have been associated with lower semen concentrations. In women, iodine is needed for egg maturation and in pregnancy: the foetus is reliant on the mother's iodine stores until eighteen weeks of gestation.

Sources: include some seaweed in your diet or take an iodine supplement. Iodine is also found in white fish and grass-fed dairy products.

Calcium

This is needed to support fertilization as well as blood clotting. It prevents vitamin D from leaching minerals from bone.

Sources: flaxseeds, sesame seeds, grass-fed dairy products, sardines and almonds.

Choline

Choline is important in the accelerated cell division that happens during pregnancy. It helps support the epigenome through methylation processes that are in charge of genetic expression during foetal development.

Sources: egg yolks, meat, legumes, yoghurt; cruciferous veggies such as cauliflower and cabbage; sunflower seeds.

Magnesium

This increases blood supply to the uterus and supports progesterone production.

Sources: buckwheat, bananas, avocados and rye.

Manganese

This can promote the breakdown of oestrogen, protecting against oestrogen dominance (see page 110).

Sources: ginger, nuts, wholegrains and broccoli.

Selenium

This mineral helps aid egg development and looks after sperm health.

Sources: Brazil nuts, garlic and eggs.

Other fertility nutrients

Coenzyme Q10

CoQ10 improves blood flow to the pelvic organs and supports mitochondrial function. In men, it's found in seminal fluid, protecting its DNA and, therefore, sperm.

Sources: liver and kidney, meat, fatty fish, nuts and seeds.

L-arginine and L-carnitine

These amino acids have been shown to improve fertility in men and women, both naturally and when using assisted techniques.

Sources: meat, dairy products, dark chocolate and nuts.

Chlorophyll

This supports tissue regeneration by promoting an increase in the red cells carrying oxygen in the blood. It can help to boost the endometrium as well as supporting developing eggs.

Sources: green vegetables and wheatgrass juice.

Inositol

This can support several signalling processes, including that of insulin and gonadotrophins, and may be especially beneficial in women with PCOS, where it can help to improve ovulation patterns.

Sources: melon, citrus fruit, sesame seeds, brown rice and beans.

N-acetyl cysteine (NAC)

This is a supplement of the amino acid cysteine, which helps to make and replenish the natural antioxidant, glutathione. It can help improve pregnancy rates by reducing the oxidative stress that damages sperm, and also helps to protect ovarian follicles. It has been shown to be especially beneficial in women with irregular ovulation (PCOS) and in those with endometriosis.

Sources: beef, turkey, eggs, fish, nuts, legumes.

Supplements

Supplements are not, and can never be, a replacement for a good diet. However, obtaining all our vitamins and minerals from food sources alone is almost impossible, given our less nutrient-rich modern diets. Lots of studies show that prenatal supplementation helps to improve fertility and minimize the risk of birth defects.

Start at least three months before conception to replenish and restore reserves, but ideally as soon as you can, for the greatest benefit.

In fact a good-quality prenatal supplement contains such a comprehensive range of vitamins and minerals that it can be used to help optimize reproductive health and general wellness, even by women who aren't necessarily looking to conceive. Supplements have been shown to improve the chance of ovulation and enhance sperm quality, reduce inflammation and increase pregnancy rates. Not all supplements are created equal. Look for the cleanest (that is, the fewest additives or, ideally, free from additives, chemicals and bulking agents), most natural and most bioavailable (absorbable) version within your budget. Carry on taking them into early pregnancy until you switch to an antenatal, which should follow the same principles.

A NOTE FOR VEGANS

Being vegan can create a mineral imbalance when it comes to your copper and zinc intake. Eating a lot of green food, including the superfoods algae and chlorophyll, can increase your copper load, which may trigger allergies and, if this is ongoing, lead to chronic inflammation. Eating plant sources of zinc, such as Brazil nuts, legumes, seeds and wholegrains, is helpful, as well as supplementing with zinc, to help balance out the copper–zinc ratio.

CHAPTER 7

Pillar 2: Exercise

Humans were built to move. You probably already know that being active boosts mood, helps sleep and is good for mental health. And that it improves your general health so much that it lengthens your lifespan. But when it comes to conception, exercise has a multitude of specific fertility effects too.

If you need a reason to pull on your trainers, read on. The list of exercise's benefits reads like a pro-conception wishlist. Not only has moderate exercise been shown to have a positive impact on pregnancy and live birth rates, but the benefits appear to be greatest in women with an endocrine or metabolic dysfunction, such as PCOS, and those with a high BMI.

Exercise increases blood flow to the reproductive organs, which can help improve the regularity of the menstrual cycle, as well as ovulation and even implantation. Regular intentional movement is thought to improve immune function and reduce inflammation, both of which increase fertility rates in women and have a beneficial effect on sperm health in men. It also potentially explains why, over time, regular exercise can help to reduce the incidence of infertility related to endometriosis, as well as the physical pain associated with this condition.

Working out has another, very fundamental benefit: it supports the health of mitochondria, the batteries that fuel each of your cells. While mitochondrial health is key to building muscle mass, it's also important in producing sex hormones. And mitochondria are instrumental in numerous key processes of the egg and sperm, such as maturation, fertilization and early embryonic development. If you're over thirty, there's more good news. Mitochondria decline in number and quality with age, but supporting mitochondrial function with exercise may help to improve egg, sperm and embryo fitness, as well as reducing the effect of ageing on egg cells. Mitochondria can adjust their volume, structure and capacity in response to exercise, and by building and maintaining muscle mass. Looking after your mitochondria through regular exercise, which in turn builds muscle mass, and through the right nutrition can help to boost fertility through all the subsequent effects mentioned above. To keep your mitochondria strong (aside from exercise), incorporate magnesium, selenium, calcium, vitamin B, copper, zinc, iron, carnitine and CoQ10 into your diet, as well as reducing refined sugars and avoiding artificial sweeteners.

The association between mitochondrial function and exercise was shown in one study, which also demonstrated an amplified effect in those who are older. Whereas a younger age group of volunteers showed a 49 per cent increase in mitochondrial capacity, an older age group demonstrated an even bigger increase of 69 per cent. Cells were encouraged to produce more mitochondrial proteins through exercise, thus increasing the anti-ageing effect. And there is another method by which exercise can have anti-ageing benefits across a range of different cells and it's related to telomeres, the capped ends of DNA that typically become compromised and shorten with age. Exercise helps to preserve telomere integrity, which declines not only with age, but also with sedentary lifestyles. It's been shown that athletic women or those who do frequent moderate exercise, have longer telomeres than women of the same age who don't. By boosting mitochondrial function, exercise also helps to reduce the chance of insulin resistance, obesity and diabetes, and slows the rate of ageing.

Irisin is a protein released by muscles during exercise, which boosts glucose uptake and increases insulin sensitivity. It also increases adipose tissue metabolism, which is closely tied in with reproductive health (see Chapter 16). Irisin has also, interestingly, been discovered in the central nervous system, as well as in the reproductive system. During the menstrual cycle, irisin levels fluctuate, increasing in the luteal phase by as much as 25 per cent. As irisin is known to inhibit oxidative stress and inflammation, having more of it may be important in achieving and maintaining pregnancy. It may also have an important role in promoting the secretion of FSH and LH from the pituitary gland, and in improving how receptive the endometrium is to the implanting embryo, especially in those with a high BMI where this receptivity may be compromised. In PCOS it may help to restore normal metabolic function and reduce the level of androgens that drive inflammation and lead to irregular ovulation. In a study of irisin-deficient mice, a negative impact was seen on their growth and development, as well as their fertility. A greater intensity of exercise helps to improve methylation and epigenetic mechanisms that promote insulin sensitivity. This, in itself, may also improve the response to ovarian stimulation in someone who requires treatment for infertility.

The fact that exercise builds your cardiovascular endurance can even make you better at sex (or at least sex for fertility!). It improves blood flow to the genitals, increases the intensity and duration of orgasm and can help prevent premature ejaculation in men. Regular exercise also minimizes the risk of pregnancy-related complications and of preterm birth.

Finally, exercise has epigenetic effects. The children of parents who exercise regularly have been shown to have different patterns of gene expression. Not only are they born healthier, but their long-term health also benefits, including their cardiovascular, metabolic and reproductive health.

Work smarter, not harder

Above all, find an exercise that you enjoy, otherwise, you won't do it! And if your workout brings you pleasure, it helps in the release of beneficial chemicals, including feel-good endorphins, dopamine and serotonin. Moving helps to rewire pain responses, such as those seen in endometriosis, and boost neuronal growth in the central nervous system, encouraging healthier neural connections and supporting neuroplasticity, which, as we saw in Part 1, is an important part of fertility.

What exercise you do should depend on any pre-existing medical conditions. On that note, please be sensible: don't exercise if you are feeling unwell or are worried about any symptoms. The advice in this chapter doesn't take into account your personal situation or fitness; speak to your doctor for specific advice if you have concerns or questions, or wish to take up new exercise or increase your exercise. That's especially true if you're having assisted reproduction procedures. When trying to get pregnant, it's best to consider how and what sort of exercise you're getting. You can exercise too much – both too long and too hard. Doing very high levels of physical activity can be so energetically intensive that it doesn't leave the body enough reserve to maintain all the necessary hormonal mechanisms for ovulation and fertilization.

Balance is the key. In studies, moderate-level exercise in moderate amounts appears to have the most beneficial effects on pregnancy rates. I usually advise my patients (both pregnant ones and those looking to conceive) to aim for 150 minutes of moderate movement a week – this is the general consensus of fitness experts and medical associations. The exercise should be spread out over the course of the week, ideally on three or more days, allowing yourself enough rest time between sessions. It is also good to vary its intensity according to your menstrual cycle (there is more advice on that in the 12-week plan).

Cortisol, the body's main stress hormone, is raised in response to exercise, but becomes chronically elevated with frequent long and intense exercise regimes and is intimately associated with many reproductive conditions, as well as the HPG axis. Ghrelin, which is an appetite-inducer, can also increase in response to stress, leaving a craving for more calorie-dense foods, so over-exercising may end up leaving you feeling hungrier and eating food that isn't necessarily good for you. This isn't to say that all high-intensity exercise is bad for you.

What exercise you do will depend on how fit you are. It's clear that a professional athlete will have different needs from someone who is usually sedentary. The upper limit is difficult to define, as it will depend on the factors mentioned earlier. But for women with a normal BMI, studies suggest that a maximum of short bursts of high-intensity exercise done intermittently (for those who are used to this form of working out) can improve blood pressure, lipid profile, insulin sensitivity and reduce levels of abdominal fat. This is true for men too; HIIT (high-intensity interval training) was found to reduce oxidative stress and inflammation, improve sperm function and promote healthy gene expression. However, if you're pregnant this does need to be adjusted accordingly and discussed with your doctor.

If you're used to being very athletic or sporty, it's possible that you'll be fine sticking to your usual programme. However, it may be a good idea to take it down a level – for example, swapping particularly intense interval training sessions, heavy weights or long runs for more moderate workouts, such as Pilates, yoga, brisk walking or swimming.

Doing more exercise may be recommended for women and men who are attempting to conceive, but who have been advised to lose weight. In women with a high BMI, exercising for longer periods has been shown to have positive benefits on fertility (but not if it's done for longer than an hour each day).

The bottom line is: find something that you love doing and just get out there. Consider it as not only an investment in your future pregnancy, but in your long-term health too.

What's your exercise intensity?

You can tell the intensity you're working out at by how you feel. But you can also use a heart-rate monitor, as the rate increases in proportion to how hard you're working. For a rough guide to your body's maximum heart rate, subtract your age from 220. *Note*: heat, caffeine and some medications can alter your heart rate. And if you suffer from any conditions, then your maximum heart rate may need adjusting.

Low intensity: if you can talk and sing without puffing, then you're exercising at a low intensity. Your heart rate is 30–50 per cent of your maximum heart rate. This can include light yoga, walking, swimming and Pilates.

Moderate intensity: if you're able to talk, but not sing, then you're exercising at moderate intensity. Your heart rate is 50–70 per cent of your maximum heart rate. This includes any activities that speed up the heart rate and breathing, but don't make you feel out of breath, such as fast yoga, cycling or dancing, as well as tennis.

High intensity: if you're unable to say more than a few words without gasping for breath, then you're exercising at a high intensity; you'll probably also be sweating. Your heart rate is 75–100 per cent of your maximum heart rate. High-intensity exercises include sprinting, heavy lifting, contact sports and CrossFit training.

Intervals: this is also called sprints or high-intensity interval training

(HIIT). You alternate between high and low intensity. High intensity increases the heart rate to near its maximum level, followed by a brief period of recovery or rest. If you're not used to exercise, then you need to condition and prepare your body first for the demands of HIIT by building up from low-intensity exercise.

TCP recommended exercises

These are some of the best forms of exercise if you're looking to conceive or are pregnant (without complications):

* **Swimming**: builds muscle tone and has cardiovascular benefits.

* **Walking and jogging**: great for the cardiovascular system, building endurance as well as reducing stress. Walking is low-impact too. Done outside, both can reduce negative emotions and fatigue. They also increase your motivation to keep exercising.

* **Resistance training**: this means using your own body weight to build muscle tone and strength, such as lunges and squats. You can also do this in yoga or Pilates, and using elastic resistance bands.

* **Yoga**: helps to reduce the stress hormone cortisol, boost mood and build muscle tone and balance as well as endurance. It also leads to the release of chemicals such as nitric oxide, which improves blood flow to the reproductive organs, tones the pelvic floor, increases sexual desire and improves orgasm. The benefits of breathwork, which is a big part of yoga, can also significantly help with stress, anxiety and general mood.

* **Dancing**: improves blood flow to the reproductive organs and offers a great aerobic workout. It's also a way to reconnect with your emotions, which will help to calm the nervous system.

❊ **Pilates**: relaxing but very strengthening, particularly for the pelvic floor. It can also help improve blood flow and improve sensation to the vagina.

❊ **Sex**: you might be surprised to see this included here! Sex is classed as moderate exercise, although sessions need to last for thirty minutes to confer any real benefits. Like dancing, having regular intercourse reduces stress and increases blood flow to the reproductive organs. But it also, of course, improves your chances of conception!

CAN I EXERCISE IF I'M HAVING ASSISTED REPRODUCTIVE TECHNOLOGY (ART)?

It used to be that during the two-week ART wait (the time between ovulation or egg collection and a pregnancy being established) people were told to stay on bed rest to increase the chances of success. But things have changed. There aren't a lot of studies, but it appears that light exercise seems to have no harmful effects on rates of implantation. In fact, doing no physical activity post-embryo transfer actually leads to a reduction in pregnancy rates. Gentle exercise during this time may also help to lift your mood and alleviate your anxiety, especially if you do it outside in daylight and in nature. Swimming isn't generally recommended post-egg collection up until the end of the two-week wait, due to the risk of infection (not to mention the chemicals), because the more open communication between your cervix and the outside world puts you at increased risk of this.

Another reason why exercise needs to be approached with caution during this time is because IVF and any other form of ovarian stimulation leads to ovarian enlargement. There's a very small but increased risk of ovarian torsion, where the ovary can twist around on its stalk, cutting off its blood supply. In particular, avoid heavy lifting, high-intensity workouts and contact sports. Always speak to your doctor about this, if you're not sure.

Male fertility and exercise

Exercise is also important for improving male fertility, but cycling is generally recognized as having negative effects on sperm parameters, which may be due to mechanical trauma to the testicles or scrotal heating. In addition, whereas moderate exercise can increase testosterone levels and boost sperm counts, too much high-intensity or impact exercise can lead to a decrease in both testosterone and thyroid levels in men. This is associated with lower sperm quality. However, exercising three to five times per week can improve sperm counts and other sperm measures in a few months, and those who practise moderate-intensity exercise show the greatest improvement. But the benefits start to decline just a week after stopping the exercise, so it's necessary to keep maintaining this.

In a similar vein to women, chronic endurance training in men is associated with suppression of the hormonal axis linking the brain with the testicles (hypothalamo–pituitary–testicular axis), which results in reduced sperm parameters, whereas those who were physically active in moderation had greater levels of antioxidant enzymes in their semen and reduced levels of DNA fragmentation. There seems to be a threshold, similar to that for women, at which the detrimental effects of too much exercise start to accumulate and affect hormonal function as well as semen. But this threshold isn't well defined at the moment, and studies remain inconclusive on the sort and amount of exercise that men should do to improve their fertility, though they are conclusive in pointing to the need for exercise to increase reproductive fitness. In general, follow the principles and advice set out above.

CHAPTER 8

Pillar 3: Stress management

CASE STUDY

Selena came to me aged thirty-five. She and her partner, Ali, had been trying to conceive for a year. They had both had investigations to look for underlying physical issues, but as none had been identified on testing, they were diagnosed with unexplained infertility.

In the appointment, Selena and Ali were quick to say they wanted to 'get on with IVF'. It's what they'd been led to believe was the next step. I asked them about the amount of stress they were experiencing in their lives, and they both denied any that they deemed to be significant. But on further questioning, it turned out they were both running their own business. Their way of relaxing in the evenings was to settle down for a glass or two of wine together. They admitted that part of this was to avoid having to discuss the emotional pain of what they were experiencing. They didn't pay a lot of attention to their nutrition; often they were too tired to cook, so they went out for dinner or ordered in.

They talked about how all their good friends had babies and children and they felt left behind. Ali confessed this was getting to him, and Selena agreed. What's more, they didn't feel they could tell their friends what they were going through, yet often felt they had to endure conversations where their friends would discuss their children and their lives as parents. Selena spent a lot of time doom-scrolling, with her Instagram feed showing her a stream of what looked like perfect families and their finely curated lives. Ali was a big worrier and admitted that he was scared children might never happen for them. He also had a strained relationship with his father, whom he didn't feel he could confide in or get the necessary emotional support from. They both felt that their only chance to conceive was with IVF.

The couple both went to bed after 11.30 p.m. most nights, not managing more than around six hours' sleep on a week-night. Neither of them thought they slept deeply. They both went to the gym regularly, with a 'go hard or go home' mentality. They were having regular sex, especially around the time of ovulation, but confessed that they often weren't emotionally present with each other or to the intimacy of sex – both being distracted by the demands of their businesses, getting pregnant or just too exhausted.

After we'd talked through their lives, I explained that I wasn't going to recommend that they did IVF at this stage. I pointed out what they could do practically to improve their natural fertility – in particular, limiting alcohol and prioritizing sleep. I advised them to shorten and tone down the intensity of their gym sessions, to mix up their routines with more restorative workouts such as Pilates and yoga and to spend more time outdoors, as well as cooking nutritionally balanced meals together. They started going for regular acupuncture sessions and tried out different meditation and breathing techniques too.

What Selena and Ali needed most was to focus on reducing stress, and to shift from constantly focusing on the future and what they were missing, towards living in the present. I asked them to write down, every day, three things they were grateful for, encouraging them to start appreciating moments of magic in their regular lives. This was part of their daily journaling, in which they began connecting with and documenting all their emotions. We discussed the impact that Ali's relationship with his dad was having on him, and the impact their close friends were having on them both as a couple. They came to the realization that having an open and honest conversation with Ali's dad and their friends about the situation they were facing would help relieve some of the stress they were carrying, and the pressure to appear in control and content. I advised them to limit time on their phones as well as exposure to the news, and to keep their work within a set number of hours. This would leave them time in the evenings to cook, to relax and to be present with each other and with themselves.

I recommended they think about how they would make space and time for a baby, and then consciously created this space in their lives, as if their baby was already there. They started a visualization meditation each evening, viewing themselves as parents and imagining their lives with a child, in as much detail as they could, including how that would feel and what they would find themselves doing differently from now.

Three months later I got a phone call to say that Selena had conceived naturally and that she had twins on the way.

When I observe patients in fertility clinics, many are rushed off their feet. They've often raced to get to the appointment on time. They have a limited time slot within which they can give the doctor only the bare minimum of details before they have to go somewhere else. The rest of their day is filled with further time pressures and demands, including the pressure of having to fund their treatment, generating even more stress, which impacts on their sleep, their food choices, their exercise and their ability to be intimate and fully present with their partner and themselves.

The non-stop nature of Selena and Ali's lives may sound familiar to you. It's nobody's fault that we live like this: society prizes achievement and rewards us when we work hard, even when it's to the detriment of our life–work balance. A major part of becoming pregnant is about surrendering, receiving, inviting, opening and being fully present to the now, rather than competing and pursuing, and it is therefore very different from how we're normally taught to believe we'll achieve what we set our minds on. Because having children has become synonymous with how we view success, when this doesn't seem to happen with ease, people are often led to believe they have failed somehow and have let themselves, and those around them, down. This sets them on a vicious circle of self-blame and judgement that generates further stress.

Why do we get stressed?

Our bodies are built to protect us from danger, which is why we have such a robust inbuilt stress or fight-or-flight response. This is part of the sympathetic nervous system, which switches on in response to any perceived danger, whether that's a lion or a professional deadline. Your neurology is pre-wired to trigger an immediate cascade of physiological changes in response to stress, increasing your breathing and heart rate, dilating your pupils, tensing your muscles and making you sweat.

Small doses of stress are valuable: they give us motivation, help us achieve our goals and perform at our best. However, long-term exposure to stress and fertility issues does not, for the simple reason it's not in your interests to conceive when the signals your body is getting indicate that you're in danger. Then your body directs its resources towards survival needs and safeguarding against anything that threatens this.

Stress and infertility

When it comes to fertility, there's enough data to suggest that we need to take stress as seriously as healthy eating and exercise. Yet it's still not something that is necessarily addressed in a medical consultation. Research has found that women with the highest levels of alpha amylase (one of the biological markers of stress in the body) have greater trouble conceiving. And women who have had an IVF cycle that didn't work have been found to have higher levels of stress-related cytokines in their blood than those who were successful. Studies also tested the blood of women who'd lost pregnancies. Those who reported high levels of stress beforehand had lower oestrogen levels, less frequent ovulation and took longer to conceive.

Stress can interfere with fertility in a multitude of ways, because it can affect all our systems, right down to the level of our genes. It can cause changes to the menstrual pattern, create hormonal imbalances, increase inflammation, pelvic pain and pain during sex, reduce blood flow to the reproductive organs, inhibit libido, prevent ovulation and negatively impact on implantation.

You've already read how interconnected all of the systems within our bodies are, and how an imbalance in one can have ripple-down effects on the others. In Chapter 2 you met the hypothalamus, the main hormonal control centre that oversees the release of several important hormones related to fertility, including oestrogen and progesterone, via the HPG (hypothalamic–pituitary–gonadal) axis.

The hypothalamus is also in charge of the stress-control system, the HPA (hypothalamic–pituitary–adrenal) axis. This is the main mechanism that keeps the sympathetic nervous system (the fight-or-flight response) activated. It controls the release of the stress hormone cortisol, which is what causes a lot of the damage to fertility.

As you read in Chapter 5, our parents' experiences, the stress our mothers were subjected to while pregnant and our childhood lives combine to create our biological response to stress. For example, studies on the children born to women who were pregnant during the 9/11 attacks showed they had higher rates of depression and anxiety and poor coping skills, compared to their peers. If the HPA axis keeps being activated – more likely in those who have inherited an easily triggered stress response – then excessive cortisol starts to cause damage through wear and tear around the body. This includes inflammation, fatigue, sugar and salt cravings, weight gain, disturbed sleep, digestive problems such as IBS, anxiety, depression and, ultimately, infertility.

However, you have control over this. Later in this chapter and in the 12-week plan you'll find ways to unwind the distorted biological wiring that you may have inherited, in order to calm your nervous system. Let's start by looking at the specific ways that stress reduces fertility.

Levels of key sex hormones go down

When under threat, the body will always divert resources to survival rather than reproduction. Both cortisol and the sex hormones are made from cholesterol, so stress leads to the body using up stores of cholesterol to make cortisol rather than sex hormones. High levels of cortisol also lead to the suppression of the key signalling hormone called gonadotrophin-releasing hormone (GnRH). The latter usually causes the ovaries to make oestrogen and progesterone (and the testes to make testosterone) but, when it's low, the brain can't effectively communicate with the ovaries, so this doesn't happen.

This has multiple knock-on effects, disturbing the monthly ebb and flow of oestrogen and progesterone. It may stop ovulation and disrupt the build-up of the lining of the womb, which depend on surges in sex-hormone levels. And as the normal effect of progesterone is to calm our nervous system, if you have low levels you may feel hyper-aroused, compounding your feelings of stress.

Oestrogen dominance

This is a continued result of hormones going awry. It gets its own section because it's so common. Often what happens under stress is that both progesterone and oestrogen will decline, but progesterone will decline more.

This can put the body into an oestrogen-dominant state. The symptoms are: fluid retention and bloating, breast tenderness, painful periods, anxiety, mood swings and depression, brain fog, abnormalities to your period such as flooding or spotting, cyclical headaches, disturbed sleep, night sweats, cystic breast disease, shorter menstrual cycles and infertility. Oestrogen dominance triggers inflammation and can increase the sensitivity of the HPA axis, intensifying the stress response.

It can also be caused, or added to, by other factors besides psychological stress, including xenoestrogens (oestrogen-mimicking substances) from the environment, impaired liver function, the combined oral contraceptive pill (COCP), a gut microbiome imbalance, constipation and a low-fibre diet. This makes the advice in the nutrition pillar (Chapter 6) and the toxin-free living pillar (Chapter 9) important if you have these symptoms.

Adverse events, in particular in childhood, have been shown to lead to inflammation, increase oestrogen dominance and increase autoantibodies.

Disruption to thyroid hormones

The thyroid is key to fertility because it has a complex feedback system with other hormones. In order to make progesterone from cholesterol, you need adequate thyroid hormones. And when progesterone levels are low, they increase the demand on your thyroid.

But if you're chronically stressed, your thyroid hormone levels may already be low, so you may end up with a double whammy of depleted thyroid stores that are unable to keep up with the demand for progesterone.

Additionally, if you don't ovulate, you won't be producing as much progesterone, and these low levels will further drive thyroid requirements. As if that wasn't enough, raised cortisol also slows down the production of thyroid hormones. Reducing stress will take the pressure off the thyroid and enable it to function better.

Inflammation

You probably think of inflammation as what happens when you are injured or have an infection. It's part of the normal short-term response of a healthy body to recruit stem cells to help injured tissue. However, your body has an inflammatory response to all kinds of stresses as well as injury, including unhealthy foods, lack of sleep, alcohol, cigarette smoke, pollution, hormone-mimicking chemicals, a sedentary lifestyle and the suppressed emotions of trauma and emotional stress. Whereas short and sharp stress can have beneficial effects on immunity and repair, stress that lasts is damaging. Chronic stress – as is often the case with unresolved emotional stress – leaves inflammation running rampant, leading to damage all over the body, which becomes hard for our bodies to repair.

This is one reason why I'm so passionate about people working on reducing their stress levels of all kinds: up to 70 per cent of unexplained infertility is thought to have an origin in inflammation and an imbalance in the immune system, yet it will so often be put down to 'unexplained' causes. Sometimes the only overt clinical signs of inner inflammation are poor egg quality, low fertilization rates and unsuccessful implantation or pregnancy loss. If we can do something to calm the inflammation before it gets to this stage, people may even avoid needing to have fertility treatment.

Poor sleep (and the sleep hormone melatonin)

Good sleep is anti-stress and pro-fertility. But we have all experienced stress that leads to sleeplessness. When you don't sleep enough, your body produces more cortisol, which makes you even more stressed, leading to further sleep deprivation.

Like stress, a lack of sleep negatively impacts on sex hormones and the womb environment and fuels inflammation. The circadian rhythm – the body's internal biological clock – responds to daylight, manages eating, body temperature and sleep cycles, but also the rhythms of your fertility-related hormones, which follow a circadian pattern of release. This rhythm influences everything from menstrual cycle regularity to follicular development, ovulation and endometrial receptivity.

The effect of lack of sleep on hormones includes unhelpful changes in progesterone and testosterone, but also reduced levels of FSH, which is associated with a shorter luteal phase of the menstrual cycle (the time between ovulation and menstruation), and reduced AMH, which is made by the ovaries and is an indicator of ovarian reserve. In fact, there seems to be an association between women who suffer from disturbed sleep and reduced ovarian reserve and lower AMH. For men, it's possible that disturbed sleep patterns can increase the production of anti-sperm antibodies, which can impact on sperm number and survival.

Studies involving shift workers – who are the classic example of a circadian rhythm that's out of sync with day and night – have shown irregular menstruation, painful periods, reduced rates of conception and an increased rate of miscarriages and endometriosis.

One key hormone here is melatonin, the pro-sleep hormone that should peak at bedtime. It's thought to have antioxidant properties that may help to improve egg and embryo quality. However, increased exposure to light at night suppresses melatonin, which can increase oestrogen levels; and when there's sleep deprivation added to this as well, your body can tip into oestrogen dominance (see page 110). This is why it's a good idea to treat both stress and sleep at the same time.

A specific stress-hormone receptor

The newest research on stress and fertility suggests a direct link between stress levels and fertility. The culprit is corticotrophin-releasing hormone (CRH), the main regulator of the HPA axis, which organizes the body's response to stress. When the HPA tells the adrenals to release stress hormones, including CRH, the receptors for CRH on various tissues are epigenetically upregulated; the upshot is that the stressful environment becomes even more sensitive to further stress.

There are CRH receptors in the central nervous system, but also all over the body. When CRH is upregulated, the brain becomes more excitable and sensitive to stress. Interestingly, CRH receptors are more prevalent in the central nervous system of women compared to men, and in particular in women over the age of forty. This can make treating stress particularly important for women of this age, who may be even more sensitive to the effects of stress.

We also now know there are local CRH receptors on reproductive organs and the placenta. For example, when researchers compared dominant follicles (containing the egg that has ovulated) that did and didn't result in a pregnancy, they found more CRH receptors on the follicle that didn't result in a pregnancy. This same pattern was also reflected in the endometrium; women who hadn't got pregnant had more CRH receptors than women who had. This suggests that CRH – and so stress – may directly influence the quality of the egg released at ovulation, as well as the process of implantation.

CRH receptors also exist on the endometriosis-related ovarian cysts (endometriomas) of patients with endometriosis. And pregnant women with pre-eclampsia appear to have a greater expression of CRH receptors, suggesting that stress could be a driver of this condition too.

All of this fits with what's been discussed in earlier chapters: individual cells respond to their immediate environment, which includes hormones, but ultimately our hormones are driven by our thought patterns and energetic signals within the body.

Increased pain

Pain is not just physical. In Chapter 5 you learned how chronic stress and pain intensify each other. This is particularly the case in people who have experienced early life trauma. If someone has a nervous system primed to be hypersensitive, as a result of trauma experienced early in childhood or in the womb, they are likely to have been conditioned to feel greater physical pain.

Interestingly there appears to be a gut–fertility connection here. The condition irritable bowel syndrome (IBS) tends to coexist with gynaecological disorders that are, in part, influenced by the effect of stress and trauma, including endometriosis. It's often referred to as a 'functional disorder', which means that medicine can't identify a physiological reason behind it. However, if you look closely at the history of many patients with this disorder, such as those with endometriosis, they tend to have a higher incidence of previous life trauma.

This isn't surprising: the brain and gut both produce and share many chemical messengers, and the gut has its own consciousness and intuition, which is why we 'feel' things in our gut. The gut is also directly affected by stress: it becomes more permeable, meaning that substances from food can spill directly into the bloodstream and cause inflammation, leading to problems with the lining of the gut, as well as constipation or diarrhoea. What starts off as psychological stress can potentially trigger further physical stress at the gut level, which then keeps the vicious cycle of physical pain and emotional distress going.

Stress and the male sex drive

In men, stress leads to lower levels of testosterone. This not only reduces sex drive, but also increases the chances of erectile dysfunction. It leads to weight gain, increases the risk of heart disease and reduces muscle mass, as well as leading to lethargy, depression and an overall reduction in well-being.

SELF-REFLECTION

In order to invite a child to come into your life, have you made the necessary space in your life for that to happen? Look at how you're living your life, and at aspects that are making you stressed and encouraging you to engage in unhealthy habits.

✳ What is your day filled with? How supportive would this be to a baby?

✳ Do you have enough time to be the parent you want to be?

✳ Would you see having a child as another job or chore?

✳ Do you currently create any space to soothe your nervous system?

✳ If you don't, how do you see yourself finding time to do this when you become a parent? Can you find ways to include self-restoration in your life?

✳ What changes can you make in your life now to become the parent you wish to be?

Dealing with stress

We all have differences in how we perceive and process stress. What may be stressful for one person isn't necessarily so for another. While we may not have control over events and circumstances, we *can* control how we respond to them. We can learn how to intentionally remodel our nervous system to respond to stress in a positive way that builds health instead of disease.

These are some of the ways you'll be dealing with stress in the 12-week plan.

Activating the vagus nerve

The gut is connected to the brain via the vagus nerve; stimulating this nerve activates the 'rest-and-digest' parasympathetic nervous system. A lot of the relaxation work and therapies you'll be doing during the 12-week plan will be working on this connection. And you'll also be working on this indirectly, by focusing on the health of your gut microbiome – the colony of bacteria that live in your gut. Getting a good balance here is key to healing a stressed nervous system (see Chapter 6).

Dealing with emotions

We may assume that positive thinking is the best policy, but the renowned psychotherapist Dr Gabor Maté says that to overcome stress we actually need to embrace the power of negative thinking. Forced positive thinking can disconnect us from emotional pain, which in turn encourages us to adopt destructive behaviours such as denial, and appearing strong.

Suppressed emotions activate a chronic level of stress that keeps your body stuck in a state of high alert and in survival mode. In his book *The Inflamed Mind*, Professor Edward Bullmore explains that inflammation in the body can affect the brain too, which then affects the production of neurotransmitters, including serotonin. This can impact on mood, sleep and appetite, and also potentially fertility, as serotonin has been shown to have a possible role in early embryo growth and development.

Avoiding uncomfortable emotions can be destructive to our bodies and brains (see Chapter 5), another reason why it's important to use a holistic approach that includes both brain and body. Your physical symptoms are signposts, directing you towards unresolved conflict, trauma or unprocessed emotional pain, to the places where you need to provide love and compassion. By facing and dealing with such emotions, you can deactivate the stress-related genetic expression that you may have inherited or acquired, and prevent further activation of stress-induced epi markers.

The key here is to embrace and accept all of your reality, including negative emotions such as rage, anger, despair and hopelessness. By doing so, you can start to lessen their long-term effect. You don't have to do this on your own: psychological support and mind–body therapy can help too. Some of the journaling prompts in the 12-week plan will support this process.

Focusing on sleep

Sleep not only resets your nervous system, but also recharges your hormones, creates natural conditions that promote detoxification and recalibrates the immune system, therefore helping to care for all the main modes of communication between the mind and the body.

You're going to work on ways to make sleep more conception-friendly. One thing that's important is to keep your circadian rhythm regular. That means getting up at around the same time each day, plenty of daylight in the morning to set your body's circadian clock and going to bed at the same time too.

It appears the magic number to aim for is seven to nine hours of sleep. The National Sleep Foundation has discovered that women who slept seven to eight hours per night were 7 per cent more likely to achieve a pregnancy than those who slept less. And those who slept eight to nine hours were 10 per cent more likely. The same is true for men too: those who slept for less than seven hours or more than nine had a 42 per cent reduction in the probability of conception.

Rhythms and rituals

We learn the importance of rhythm as a self-soothing mechanism in the womb, where we're exposed to the cadence of our mother's beating heart and the surrounding vibrations. Later, as adults, the rhythms that match this early experience feel soothing, because we associate them with feeling safe. This is why breathing techniques and tapping, as well as drumming or singing, can be so effective at making us feel better and calmer. The natural cadence in each of these helps to regulate our nervous system from a state of alertness and vigilance to one of rest and restoration. During the 12-week plan you'll develop a regular repertoire of rituals you can call on to help you to self-regulate whenever you need to. And performing rituals together with other people has been shown to lead to a synchronization of brain activity, which helps to regulate and calm the nervous system through the interconnectedness that we feel.

Mindfulness as medication

Meditation is anti-stress. Practising mindful meditation helps us tune in with what we're feeling, connect our emotions with how our body feels and deepen the bond we have with our body. It helps us to face and feel negative emotions such as fear, worry and guilt and to heal emotional pain. And it can help reveal our inner strength, increasing our capacity for self-love and our compassion for others.

One of its main mechanisms is that, when we meditate, we change our brains over time. Specifically, we restructure the prefrontal cortex, the part of the brain that is involved in self-control and concentration. As a result, we're better able to manage emotions and access happiness. Regular meditation has been shown to reduce pain and reliance on painkillers. And it's also been shown to reduce inflammation and slow down ageing by keeping telomeres longer. Researchers have found that even in those new to meditation, close to a thousand different genes were positively impacted by its effect.

Short, sharp stresses

Small intermittent bursts of stress, such as cold water and high-intensity exercise, can work to counter the effects of chronic stress, through a process called hormesis. They can lead to repair of cell damage and of DNA, as well as neutralization of oxidative stress and associated free radicals, an increase in the production of mitochondria, a reduction in inflammation, a boost to natural detoxification, a reduction in insulin resistance and a reduced risk of cancer. Many of these same processes are also involved in promoting fertility, so their benefits extend to improving reproductive potential. And they may also help us to adapt better to other stressors of the negative sort – a process called cross-adaptation. Ideally such stresses should be done when we feel relaxed, to future-proof against stressful situations that may come later and to build resilience. Avoiding doing them in the second half or luteal phase of the cycle is important, as this is when we're most sensitive to cortisol and when our body is most susceptible to stress. You'll be doing some short, sharp stresses in the 12-week plan.

Activating the heart–brain connection

The heart does more than simply pump blood – it's a 'little brain'. It contains specialized cells called sensory neurites that behave in a similar way to brain cells; they can process, memorize, perceive and respond, as well as store emotion. The heart has an electromagnetic field that is thought to be 5,000 times greater than the brain's, and it has a profound impact on the rest of the body all the way down to our cells. The heart also has its own neural network that sends more signals to the brain than the brain does to the heart, and its one of the first organs to form. The highest state of well-being is when your heart, mind and emotions are in energetic alignment and cooperation, which the US HeartMath Institute has dubbed 'Heart Coherence'. In this state, we can self-regulate and deal effectively with stress.

When the nervous system is dysregulated, it impairs the brain's ability to self-regulate and to access higher cognitive functions. It also changes heart rate variability (HRV) – the variation in time between each heartbeat – so that HRV is a good measurement of how stressed we are, where stress is correlated with lower levels of variability, and higher variability relates to greater resilience.

We can literally rewire the circuit between our heart and our brain towards Heart Coherence by cultivating positive emotions such as compassion and love, as well as projecting gratitude and happiness, which lead to the release of neurochemicals that support healing and well-being. It's been shown that doing this increases HRV, a sign of true physiological relaxation. With such a powerful effect on the entire energetic and physical body, it's no wonder the heart chakra is often considered the most important chakra. You'll be tapping into its power during the 12-week plan, when you do the core heart-chakra meditation.

Time in nature

This isn't strictly a therapy, but it acts like one. Our nervous systems evolved to relax in natural settings. In fact there are now more than 100 scientific studies that show the beneficial effects of nature on human health and well-being. Go outside for twenty minutes in a green space and you'll feel the relaxation response kick in: it's rapid and innate. In the 12-week plan you'll introduce more nature into your life. It doesn't have to be a full immersion in the countryside. It's been shown that even small elements of nature – plants and flowers placed in a hospital room – reduce activation of the stress response and even increase pain tolerance.

Stress is an unavoidable part of life, but when we practise adaptive rather than maladaptive strategies to help us deal with it, we can cultivate an internal landscape geared towards health rather than disease, and so lessen the impact stress may have on our future children.

CHAPTER 9

Pillar 4: Toxin-free living

Although our lives may be technologically advanced, to improve our fertility we need to adopt a more natural way of living.

Every day we're exposed to a whole range of chemicals. Take the air we breathe. Particularly in cities, it can be polluted with lead, mercury, cadmium, benzene, ammonia and formaldehyde. What about the tap water we drink? This too can contain chemicals, including a group of industrial chemicals called PFAS (Perfluoroalkyl and Polyfluoroalkyl Substances). These are often called 'forever chemicals' because of how long they last in the environment.

The chemicals we encounter can have a profound effect, influencing and interacting with our genes. This is concerning for preconception because our bodies can become repositories for them. The chemicals can accumulate in fatty tissues, including the reproductive organs, and can pass into the placenta and breast milk. Some have been linked with the development of infertility, as well as with cancer and birth defects, and some of their effects can be magnified down future generations.

But there is very little regulation concerning most of these chemicals. While packets of cigarettes warn that smoking causes disease, we don't have similar labels regarding common food additives and ingredients containing chemicals that studies have linked with diseases, including MSG, aspartame, nitrates, GMO and some food colourings.

What do chemicals do to our bodies?

The effects of many of these chemicals on our bodies remain largely under-investigated and undiagnosed. We do know that some chemicals mimic and bind to the same receptors as our own hormones. The Endocrine Society, a global organization of endocrine clinicians and investigators, has warned about the dangers to fertility and human health if we continue to leave endocrine disruptors unregulated in our population.

For example, environmental oestrogens, or xenoestrogens, mimic oestrogen by binding to the same receptor sites, disrupting how our own oestrogen works in our bodies. These fake hormones may be contributing to changes including male breast development, penis size and an earlier average onset of periods in girls, which is down from the age of eleven to nine.

There's been a worldwide drop in fertility of 50 per cent between 1960 and 2015. The reality is that many women and men in their most potently fertile years are less fertile than their grandparents were in their mid-thirties. In men in Western countries, sperm counts and testosterone levels have gone down drastically over the last forty years. Erectile dysfunction is rising, along with testicular cancer, and libidos are falling.

In women, premature ovarian ageing (the ovaries stop functioning as they should, before the age of forty) appears to be on the rise, having increased from around 20 per cent in 2004 to just under 30 per cent in 2011. Conditions such as PCOS, endometriosis and tubal-factor infertility, which are influenced by the environment and the epigenome, are on the rise too. Cutting down on exposure to toxins is one of the pillars of TCP because before and during pregnancy are the most important times to act. The placenta doesn't prevent a lot of chemicals from reaching the foetus; the result is that what the mother is exposed to – from the air she inhales, to the products she applies – can be absorbed by the baby. In fact the average placenta has been shown to contain more than 200 exogenous chemicals, and breast milk may contain even more. However, there is a lot that can be done to reduce this exposure and its subsequent potential effects.

One of the key times is during the first trimester, when the baby's sexual organs, driven by the presence or absence of testosterone, begin to differentiate and develop. This is when they are most sensitive to external influence. Androgen-blocking chemicals may lead to lower sperm counts, lower testosterone, an increase in undescended testicles and testicular cancer, and abnormalities with the penis.

Chemicals can affect not only the health of our eggs and sperm, but also the long-term health of future generations. The womb environment is crucial in determining a child's health and reproductive ability later in life too. Although the impact of some of these chemicals can start off small, it can become magnified over generations. For example, it's been shown that phthalates from plastics can not only affect embryo quality, but can negatively affect the fertility of the baby that's yet to be born too. The older we are, the lower our ability to naturally detox from many of these chemicals, and the longer the ovaries and testicles spend being exposed to their potential harmful side-effects.

These chemicals also affect our microbiome: the 140 trillion bacteria that form our internal ecosystem. When healthy, the microbiome is one of the ways in which we neutralize toxins. But over-exposure to some of these chemicals can compromise its make-up and its functioning.

If you've been diagnosed with unexplained infertility, or in fact any form of infertility, it may be a good idea to consider being tested for your toxin exposure or subsequent nutrient deficiencies, and how well your body is metabolizing any toxins, as this could provide some important insights. Some functional doctors, nutritionists and naturopaths provide these tests. More targeted treatment can then be undertaken to correct this and to optimize the conditions not only for your fertility and health, but also for the health of your future children.

Leading a toxin-free lifestyle

Living a totally toxin-free life just isn't possible, however committed you are. But it's worth cleaning up the toxins that you can: think of making the necessary lifestyle changes before and during pregnancy as like preparing good soil for growth. This pillar isn't about overhauling your entire household. It's about small, liveable changes that you can introduce during the 12-week plan.

Once you've learned to recognize the chemical names, the suggested changes will become simple. (When you're not sure about ingredients or additives, the Chemical Maze app and others are a good place to check.)

Here are some key areas where you can begin to detoxify your life.

Personal care

* **Start buying clean personal-care products**: find products that don't contain the chemicals listed below or replace them with natural alternatives, such as oils as a moisturizer instead of creams or making your own face-mask. Look for an aluminium-free deodorant. Chemicals to avoid are: phthalates, parabens, benzyl alcohol, phenoxyethanol, triclosan, benzoic acid, petroleum-based polymer derivatives (PEGs), benzophenone, talc, paraffin, petroleum and mineral oil, lead, toluene, butylated hydroxyanisole (BHA) and butylated hydroxytoluene (BHT), cadmium, musks, siloxanes, ammonia, sodium laureth sulphate and resorcinol.

* **Don't take unnecessary medication**: when used over long periods of time, even paracetamol can be damaging to sperm and can increase the time required to achieve pregnancy.

* **Change your sanitary protection**: the vagina is one of the most sensitive parts of the body to chemicals, with a large surface area and high absorption rates. Whatever goes inside can have a major effect. Synthetic fibres can contain plastic chemicals, and you also want to avoid pesticide residues, so switch to organic and pure-cotton tampons and towels. Even better, as it can be reused, try organic cotton period underwear.

* **Be mindful of hair dyes**: many women worry about colouring their hair while trying to become pregnant or when pregnant. Hair salons and even supermarkets now offer lower-toxin hair dyes. Try to minimize the dye's contact with the scalp if you can, by opting for balayage instead of highlights, for example.

* **Work on your dental hygiene**: floss regularly and book in regularly at the hygienist for a clean. Women with gum disease take longer to get pregnant, and an overgrowth of

gum bacteria can affect sperm too. See your dentist if you are worried about mercury tooth fillings (too many of these may impact on the liver's detoxification process) and consider having them replaced. Replace regular toothpaste with a more natural one, along with a mouthwash that doesn't contain alcohol, artificial sweeteners, flavours or colours.

* **Don't use antibacterial soap**: antibacterials kill off both good and bad bacteria, adding to antibiotic resistance, and can also create harmful chemicals when they react with the chlorine in tap water.

* **Avoid microwave meals and plastic bottled water**: microplastics may be able to get into the heart, brain and lungs of unborn children and lead to adverse effects on health.

FOUR DETOX HELPERS

1. **Take regular baths with Epsom salts** to help draw out impurities that you may have accumulated. And sweat at least a couple of times a week in a sauna or by exercising (if you are pregnant or having fertility treatment, avoid excessive sweating).

2. **Invest in a regular massage or get your partner to give you one.** Give yourself a daily two-minute session of dry body-brushing. These techniques keep the lymphatic as well as the circulatory system moving, which is important for detoxing.

3. **Incorporate regular vegetable-based green smoothies into your diet,** because these foods can help bind to various toxins and reduce their load on the body.

4. **Eat food rich in diindolylmethane (DIM),** such as broccoli, avocados and cauliflower, which binds excess oestrogen in the body and prevents its absorption. Eating avocados can also help balance out any excess oestrogen.

Kitchen

* **Replace aluminium, copper and non-stick pots and pans with enamel, cast iron and stainless steel**: some non-stick chemicals have been associated with foetal growth defects and oestrogen imbalances. If you do use a non-stick pan, use a wooden spoon to avoid scraping the surface.

* **Replace plastic cooking utensils, jugs, bowls and chopping boards with wood, glass or stainless steel.**

* **Stop buying and storing food in plastic**: and in particular stop heating food in plastic. Use glass, metal or ceramic containers instead. Bisphenol A (BPA), butylated hydroxyanisole (BHA), polyvinyl chloride (PVC) and phthalates are all types of xenoestrogens found in plastics. And they can leach into food and water, especially when heated or at very cold temperatures.

* **Buy from farmers' markets and zero-waste refill shops to avoid packaging**; at home, rinse fruit and veg before using.

* **Reduce the amount of processed, takeaway and even restaurant food that you eat**: these all increase the chance of plastic contaminants reaching your food through packaging and gloves.

* **Invest in a water filter**: keep well hydrated throughout the day, as water will help the natural detoxification processes in your body. Unfiltered tap water contains chlorine as well as traces of toxic metals, medications (including the pill), aluminium and personal-care products. Ideally buy a filter that is glass or stainless steel rather than plastic. And definitely avoid drinking from plastic bottles!

Home

❋ **Think natural when it comes to materials**: whether it's your hairbrush or the furniture in your home, opt for wood instead of plastic. Use sponges and cloths made from natural instead of synthetic fibres, cotton or linen tea towels, and paper (hemp or beeswax) for wrapping food instead of aluminium or cling film.

❋ **Buy cleaning products that are free from synthetic chemicals and scents**; or create your own using natural ingredients.

❋ **Avoid synthetically fragranced air fresheners and synthetically fragranced candles**; instead, use beeswax or natural wax candles.

❋ **Convert to natural laundry detergent that's free from phthalates, phosphates, petroleum and artificial dyes**: these are gentler on the skin, with a much lower chance of causing irritation and allergies.

❋ **Quarantine or ventilate new curtains, furniture, mattresses, bedding and carpets**: volatile organic compounds (VOCs) are found in many common household items. They are not water-soluble and therefore they accumulate in fatty tissue, where their effect can last for many years.

❋ **Replace carpets with wooden flooring or ceramic tiling**: this makes it easier to minimize dust, which contains VOCs.

❋ **Leave outdoor shoes at the door and swap to slippers**, to avoid bringing pollutant-laden dirt and dust inside.

❋ **Choose lead-free dinnerware**: lead can hang around in our bodies for two decades. It displaces calcium and can get into the bones and heart, as well as into the brain. Antique porcelain and clay dinnerware is prone to contamination.

⁂ **Decorate with paints and varnishes that are marked as non-toxic and natural:** these have low VOCS.

⁂ **Keep potted plants in your home, as they can help to convert VOCs;** helpful plants include bamboo palm, ivy, moss, rubber plant and fern.

⁂ **Wear clothes made from natural fibres:** cotton, wool, silk and linen. Buy less but higher-quality, so that they last longer, and buy (and sell or donate) second-hand. Synthetic fabrics not only contain synthetic chemicals, but when they are washed or dried they leach microplastics, which end up in the water and soil. If you do buy synthetic items, choose those made from recycled fibres.

⁂ **If it's hot, before you get into your car, open the windows and doors so that the car can ventilate,** then drive with the windows closed and the air conditioning on, to avoid the chemicals and heavy metals from traffic, such as benzene, carbon monoxide and lead.

CHECK THE LABEL

This goes for food, but also for clothes and face creams. Just because a product says it's 'natural' doesn't mean it's all-natural. If it says 'organic', check it's been certified. As a general rule of thumb, the longer the list of ingredients, the greater the chance the product isn't natural.

Electromagnetics

We're surrounded by electric and wireless signals wherever we go, from our phones to Wi-Fi and TV. The evidence isn't conclusive, but there is an increasing concern about their potential harmful effects – for example, interfering with the body's natural electromagnetic circuits. This could potentially affect egg and sperm quality, as well as causing generalized health issues, such as tiredness, headaches, brain fog, irritability, thyroid issues and heart palpitations.

* **Minimize your exposure to Wi-Fi** by switching your router off at night.

* **Use the loudspeaker when speaking on your mobile,** rather than bringing it close to your head.

* **Keep your mobile phone encased in a protective cover** to reduce heat radiation.

* **Don't keep your phone in a pocket,** to avoid any radiation that could impact upon eggs and/or sperm.

* **Switch to incandescent light bulbs where possible;** fluorescent and compact fluorescent bulbs (CFLs) contain a small amount of mercury, which is a neurotoxin. LED bulbs also contain heavy-metal toxins, including lead.

* **Avoid using a microwave,** as older ones can emit radiation. But even a newer one will alter the chemical bonds in food, producing free radicals while destroying antioxidants and vitamins.

The trouble with smoking

If you need motivation to give up smoking, then trying for a baby is the best reason of all. In men, smoking damages sperm, reducing their number, motility and adversely affecting their shape. It also increases damage to DNA, reduces testosterone and can lead to erectile dysfunction. In women, it increases the time taken to get pregnant, both with and without IVF; it also reduces egg reserves and leads to an earlier menopause. On top of that, it raises the risk of chromosomal abnormalities, and miscarriage rates are higher in smokers, as is the incidence of ectopic pregnancy.

It's not just cigarettes. Regular marijuana use is also associated with adverse effects on sperm and increased risk of miscarriage. There's evidence that e-cigarettes and vaping increase infertility too, although the data on this is still preliminary.

As you can see, there are many inexpensive ways in which you can avoid some of the most common toxins, even if you can't eliminate them altogether. These are not only better for you and your future baby, but also for our planet. They may seem like small changes, but when practised over longer periods of time, their benefits can be significant and cumulative.

CHAPTER 10

Pillar 5: Sex and relationships

The very fact that IVF exists creates a mechanistic view of the body, as fertilization can now take place without even having sex. This is perpetuated by fertility medicine too: the only part of sex that most medical professionals will tend to ask about is how often you're having sex and whether there is any pain or difficulty with erection or ejaculation. This mechanistic view of the body treats sex as purely functional, which is ironic, because anyone who's tried to become pregnant for a long time will tell you that having sex with the sole purpose of conception *can* eventually become functional – a chore rather than a pleasure, and far removed from what it used to be when you and your partner first started.

This chapter covers some useful information that you need to know about the sort of sex that is conducive to conception. But the main point is: sex is so much more than sperm-meets-egg. Regular sex, or masturbation if you're single, provides a long list of biological and psychological benefits, a lot of which can help conception too. Sex boosts mood and improves mental health, reduces stress, increases intimacy, improves your relationship with your partner and the one you have with yourself. It can restore energetic balance and help you connect with your spirituality. It helps to boost blood flow to the reproductive organs, improves the chances of ovulation and helps to regulate the menstrual cycle. It can in some cases be even more therapeutic than medication, helping to relieve tension, reduce menstrual cramps and other sources of pain, improve bladder control, lower blood pressure, improve heart health and immunity and lead to better sleep. Oh, and did I forget to mention it feels good too?

In fact a lot of this chapter is about why pleasure is one of the most important dimensions of sex for conception. Sexual pleasure is not hedonistic; it's part of our hardwiring. It's something each of us is set up to receive, and can experience. The clitoris has 8,000 nerve endings and the penis has 5,000, and these feed information directly to the brain. Pleasurable sex releases feel-good neurochemicals and hormones that create an internal environment that favours conception. This chapter explores how, if sex currently feels like something to be ticked off the to-do list, it can instead become a life-enhancing turn-on.

When and how often do I need to have sex?

These are the questions I'm most often asked. And the most important thing I want to get across is to have sex often, throughout your cycle. This advice may go against what you've been told, which is to have sex during the 'fertile window'.

It's true that the fertile window, as shown on the diagram below, is important. The science of ovulation has revealed that the vast majority of pregnancies are conceived during this time, and only a tiny percentage before and after. This diagram presupposes that you have a 28-day cycle (and are ovulating); see below if your cycle is shorter/longer. You'll find a key to tracking your cycle in the 12-week plan too.

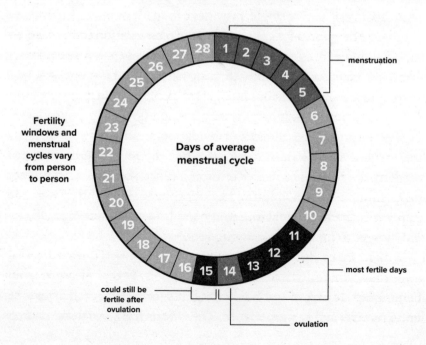

HOW LONG DOES OVULATION LAST?

menstruation

Fertility windows and menstrual cycles vary from person to person

Days of average menstrual cycle

could still be fertile after ovulation

most fertile days

ovulation

❋ At the beginning of each cycle (Day 1 on this chart) several follicles from both ovaries begin to grow. Eventually one of them usually develops into the dominant follicle that matures the egg that has ovulated in the middle of the cycle (Day 14 on this chart).

❋ The egg can be fertilized anywhere from six to twenty-four hours after ovulation. And sperm can survive for up to five days in cervical mucus. There need to be enough sperm arriving in the right place in this lead-up to ovulation and on the day of ovulation.

❋ This makes a roughly six-day period in each menstrual cycle when pregnancy is possible, depending on when ovulation occurs. This is the fertile window; it starts at Day 10 of your cycle, but can be slightly earlier or later, if your cycles are short or long, respectively.

❋ The greatest chance of fertilization is on the actual day of ovulation. You can monitor your own signs of ovulation or use an ovulation-predictor device (see the 12-week plan), but please don't become obsessed by it!

❋ However, the timing of ovulation can vary (as can the length of cycle). And so the most important time to have regular intercourse is during the first half of your cycle, which is called the follicular phase. That is, Days 1–14, but especially on Days 10–14.

So why do I advise having regular sex all month? First, research suggests it's possible to ovulate more than once per cycle! A 2003 study gave daily ultrasound scans to fifty women, all of whom had regular menstrual cycles. It found that two out of three had at least two waves of follicles developing in their ovaries. It's still unusual to ovulate more than once, because the luteinizing hormone (LH) surge that prompts ovulation usually occurs only once in a cycle, but it's possible. Multiple ovulations may be more common in women who are older, in women with a family history of twins and shortly after stopping hormonal birth control, due to higher FSH (follicle-stimulating hormone).

There's an even more compelling reason to have sex all month: the positive effect that sex has on the immune system. Women who had regular and frequent sex were found to have higher levels of cytokines, chemicals that prime the immune system in preparation for pregnancy, reducing the risk of sperm and embryos being rejected. For men, regular sex can help improve sperm quality and motility too.

Research suggests that regular contact with seminal fluid may prime an optimum environment for conception and stimulate ovulation. In mice, it's been shown that regular sex leads to beneficial epigenetic changes in the Fallopian tubes, and anti-inflammatory immune changes that boost the chances of implantation too. Regular sex may even have a positive knock-on effect on the health of the pregnancy, the mother and the baby. For example, in humans it's been shown that women who've had less intercourse before conceiving are more likely to develop pregnancy disorders such as pre-eclampsia and gestational diabetes.

While you may be thinking, 'Oh no, now I've got to have *more* sex to get pregnant', please listen to your own body. Instead of being rigid about sex during the fertile window, try relaxing into more spontaneous sex throughout the month, *including* the window. There will be days when you simply won't feel like having sex, and that's okay. Don't feel under pressure. As you and your partner become healthier through using TCP, you'll find a natural side-effect will be an increase in libido. And remember: regular sex is better for your stress levels and intimacy, both of which improve the chances of successful conception.

The brain is a sex organ too

Forcing yourself to have sex in order to get pregnant is stressful. And when your body is under stress (as you saw in Chapter 8), it's not conducive to getting pregnant. It's interesting that the word matrix in Latin means the womb, reflecting the capacity it has to process information from the outside. Stress interferes with neurotransmitters, muscle relaxation and blood-vessel engorgement, which can lead to problems in experiencing arousal. When you are chronically stressed, the epigenome of the vagina can change too, leading to changes in the tissue that may influence sexual response.

The vaginal epigenome can also be affected by other factors, such as your underwear, sanitary products and semen. Experiments on fruit flies – which make good models for human genetics – have shown that the semen from a male fruit fly can trigger epigenetic changes in the female, affecting fertility and libido, but also immunity, as well as sleep patterns and egg and embryo development. Although studies have yet to be done in humans, your partner may be influencing your long-term health and fertility via sex.

You absorb some semen through the vaginal wall, and as this contains FSH, LH, oestrogen, testosterone and prostaglandins, it impacts on your internal hormonal environment and neurotransmitters. This may be why studies find that women who have regular unprotected intercourse with their partner tend to live longer and healthier lives (provided there are no STDs). You may be helping to look after your male partner's health too; we know that female neuropeptides can help protect the prostate gland.

PAIN DURING SEX

Painful sex, or dyspareunia, is very common. Around one-third of women experience it at any given time, and most don't see their doctor about it. Deep dyspareunia can be due to a pelvic condition such as endometriosis or an ovarian cyst or fibroid, and sometimes from the effect of previous childbirth. But this, or superficial dyspareunia, which is pain before penetration, can sometimes be due to emotional causes. When women are stressed, it can interfere with muscle relaxation and blood-vessel engorgement, leading to problems experiencing arousal. Pelvic-floor muscles can store the emotions and tension from previous negative sexual experiences too. Both physical and verbal negative experiences trigger the stress circuit, tipping the body into survival mode. This increases the perception of pain, which can contribute to painful sex and conditions such as vulvodynia or vaginismus. Chronic stress also changes the epigenome of the vagina and this can influence sexual response (see Chapter 19).

The pleasure–conception connection

Being aroused can provide profound surges of oestrogen, which is particularly important for conception in women with low levels – that is, those who are chronically stressed or older. In fact enjoying sex, the bodily contact of sex and having an orgasm (or more than one!) can have significant anti-stress benefits. Don't let this stress you out about achieving an orgasm, but do turn your attention towards improving your own capacity for pleasure, and the relationship with your partner (if you have one) and yourself.

The starting point for pleasure is always having a sexual relationship with yourself. Being able to feel pleasure helps you to connect deeper into yourself and your own feelings. Masturbation puts you in touch with who you are and expands your understanding of pleasure. Many of us weren't told or taught about masturbation openly and so have an aversion both to discussing and doing it. In fact research suggests that being open with teenage girls is as protective as being told about contraception, but rather than preventing pregnancy, it stops the shame and guilt that can develop around sex when young women aren't informed about sexual pleasure.

During pleasurable sex you release the feel-good hormones dopamine and serotonin, plus those boosts of oestrogen and testosterone, as well as a spike in oxytocin, which is often called the 'love hormone' or 'bonding hormone'. Oxytocin has a brilliant side-effect: it reduces cortisol levels and so helps regulate our stress response, which has a beneficial effect on sex hormones. Sex boosts production of the hormone prolactin, which puts the uterus into a state of receptivity.

Nitric oxide, which is produced by blood vessels in response to arousal, increases blood flow to the sexual organs; the clitoris and erectile tissue in the vulva area engorge, the vagina lubricates and elongates and the uterus and cervix lift. These changes help to draw sperm closer to the uterine opening. They also lead to even more pleasure, including the clitoris pushing against the front wall of the vagina to create the G-spot.

Sex is like a chemical conversation between two bodies: the cells of your reproductive system are constantly sending out hormones and other signals, and receiving them from your partner too. Studies suggest that we swap chemicals called neuropeptides during sex, which increase female arousal; pre-clinical studies suggest they may enhance the uterine and Fallopian-tube environment too, favouring conception. Research from Monash University in Melbourne, Australia, suggests that chemicals released by the ovary, including progesterone, guide the sperm to the egg and help activate sperm to penetrate it too; essentially, the egg chooses the sperm.

The epigenetic concoction of neuropeptides and hormones during intercourse may also encourage anatomical changes in the curvature of the Fallopian tube, to help guide sperm on their way to the egg. Finally, the pheromones in your natural scent – as well as being attractive to your partner – may enhance sperm–egg interaction, because both testes and sperm have olfactory (scent) receptors. This helps boost the chances of conception around the time of ovulation, when pheromones are at their peak.

So pleasure, and the capacity to experience pleasure during sex, matters because it effectively and epigenetically dictates how favourable the conditions are for conception to occur.

Is orgasm important for conception?

The Greek physician Hippocrates, who lived 2,400 years ago, is considered to be the father of modern medicine. He believed that both men and women needed to climax for conception to occur, 'bursting forth seed'. Although having an orgasm isn't *technically* necessary for conception, it may boost your chances.

An orgasm creates a mechanical suction effect, sucking the sperm through the cervix towards the Fallopian tubes. Orgasming potentially helps a woman retain 15 per cent more semen in her uterus. And the release of oxytocin post-orgasm creates uterine peristalsis – a series of small contractions that helps move the sperm towards the egg.

Again, masturbation is key here, as it helps you to know what works for you and increases your potential for orgasm. Be careful about using vibrators too often to help, though. Depending on a vibrator can lead to problems becoming aroused without one, as it can lead to desensitization. To find new ways to orgasm, explore stimulation not only of the clitoris through touch, but of the whole of the front vaginal wall and deeper tissue, because orgasm can be achieved through stimulation of these different points, and not simply the clitoris and G-spot. Try to have a longer build-up to orgasm; this not only creates a favourable hormonal environment for orgasm, but also conception, as described above. The same is true for men, as a build-up will increase testosterone; for women, it will bring the cervix closer to the penis.

WHAT POSITION IS BEST FOR CONCEPTION?

You may have heard that lying on your back helps improve the chances of sperm reaching the egg, or that afterwards you should put your legs up the wall or pedal your legs in the air. This is based on something called the 'poleaxe hypothesis', which says that lying down after sex allows ejaculated sperm to travel more quickly up the vaginal canal towards the egg.

Some studies done on women having intrauterine insemination (IUI), where sperm is put into the uterus (see Chapter 14), have shown that lying down for fifteen minutes after the procedure may increase pregnancy rates. However, a 2017 meta-analysis that looked at several IUI studies didn't find this benefit. Bear in mind that studies can't replicate what goes on with natural conception, when orgasm and stimulation can have added benefits.

Sperm travels fast after ejaculation, arriving at the Fallopian tube anywhere between five and fifteen minutes afterwards, no matter what position you're in. Giving them a head-start of a few millimetres is unlikely to make a big difference.

The upshot is: there isn't a scientifically validated or approved position in which to have sex. Some women may dislike certain positions or find them painful. Figuring out what suits you best and is most comfortable will help reduce stress, and it's this that will ultimately improve your chances of conception, rather than the position itself.

Infertility and relationships

Sex is powerful on many levels, and is the most potent anti-ageing tool we have. We already know that it can help increase lifespan and keep people healthier for longer. Ancient Incan traditions didn't see sex as merely for procreation, but as an act of healing. And I support that view. It's the most powerful creative force we have access to, not only for conceiving a child, but also for tapping into your creative power when it comes to projects and other accomplishments in the world. It connects us with the truth of who we are, opens our heart centre and restores energetic balance by activating our other energetic centres (chakras), which means that sex can be a deeply healing and emotional experience. That post-coital glow people have after sex reflects this multitude of internal benefits.

In a safe, nurturing relationship, sex can also help us to become more embodied, while it deepens the bond with ourselves and our partner. In spiritual terms, when a man penetrates and touches the cervix, this can lead to the woman's mind relaxing and her heart opening, so that each person renews and regenerates the other. The G-spot is energetically connected via a meridian to the pineal gland, the site of the third-eye or brow chakra. And so having sex can bring us closer to spiritual encounters, raising our level of awareness and consciousness and helping us to more fully embody our body, mind and soul.

However, when you feel stress and anxiety around becoming pregnant, it can compromise the positive impact of sex, because of the sex organs being directly wired to the brain. When we don't experience pleasure during sex, it can lead to us withholding our feelings from our partner; we can become disconnected and eventually start to pull away from them. Goal-oriented sex puts pressure on both of you. It can affect the relationship with your partner and the relationship you have with yourself. Your partner may feel helpless or inadequate because they can't fix the fact of not getting pregnant and, when they see you in distress, they may shift into problem-solving mode, which can become even more disconnecting. It becomes a vicious cycle: the stress around not getting pregnant leads to sex that isn't conducive to allowing conception to happen, which contributes to further stress, which leads to a reduction in libido that disconnects you further from pleasure and from yourself, as well as your partner . . . and on it goes.

Be mindful of the consciousness you bring to sex. Share how you're feeling with your partner, and what emotions are coming up for you. Help them to feel safe in expressing to you how they feel. If there are emotional issues that you haven't discussed with your partner, it can have an impact on your energetic body and make it harder to become pregnant (see Chapter 3 on how the energetic body is closely related to our physical body via the chakras and meridians).

When you want to talk to your partner about sex, or explore what's happening in your relationship, or say where you feel your needs weren't met, do it when both of you are not feeling stressed or tired. Then your abilities to listen and hold a compassionate space will be much greater and less judgemental.

In times of stress, be aware that you both bring your own patterns from childhood and past experiences. For example, if you're triggered by your partner, then old feelings of abandonment, shame or dishonour may arise. Recognize that your initial reaction is your preconditioned survival mechanism, and avoid the temptation to react by blaming, judging or criticizing your partner. See if you can both engage in finding solutions together and in being open and honest about how you're feeling.

Our bodies carry the imprints of all our previous sexual encounters, which condition our neurological, immune and hormonal systems. Releasing and healing the trauma we're holding onto is so important in being able to cultivate a relationship of trust with our bodies. This is why doing the work set out earlier in this book (in Chapter 5) and in the 12-week plan will not only benefit you, but also your relationship. Seeing a counsellor – alone or together – to deal with difficult emotions from not being pregnant, or from any other relationship strains, can help you to heal and process stressful life circumstances and the difficult emotions of infertility. Counselling may improve not only the relationship you have with your partner, but also with yourself.

When it comes to sex itself, it may help to think of it as starting way before you get into bed. Creating anticipation helps boost arousal and all its positive benefits, increasing the chance of orgasm. So build up to sex during the day by exchanging messages and flirting. You can do foreplay alone, but not only through sexual arousal: self-care and pleasure of any kind counts, whether it's doing something you love, watching a beautiful sunset, walking barefoot outside on the grass or buying yourself flowers: all of these will help to prime you for a better sexual response. We are wired to process pleasure, and a physical or erogenous response doesn't need to be through sexual means alone.

Spending some time apart, in anticipation of sex, can be helpful too: newness increases the production of dopamine, which creates a surge of testosterone for men and of oestrogen for women. In bed, exploring erogenous zones, taking time and not rushing the experience are the best way to create the hormonal cascade that is beneficial for conception. Begin by seeking pleasure within yourself, and then with your partner. There's more on ways to do this below, and in the 12-week plan. I hope that any sexual experience you have from now on leads you to greater emboldening, a new positive consciousness, self-love and respect for your incredible body and its capacity for joy, pleasure and creation.

Things to do for more satisfying sex and a closer relationship

There is more on this in the 12-week plan, but this is a good place to start.

* **Cultivate a good relationship with your vagina**: this is something that never gets mentioned, yet it's a vital part of building self-confidence and well-being; 44 per cent of women can't tell what the vagina is, on an anatomical diagram, and even more say they can't bear to look at their own vulvas. Learn to appreciate the uniqueness of yours, its folds and curvatures, accepting any asymmetries as part of being normal. Practise doing this with a hand-mirror, as part of your regular self-care. At the same time examine the clitoris, the inner and outer labia and vaginal wall, and look for any spots, soreness or pain, bumps, itching, redness or change in colour, or any other alterations.

* **Speak words of compassion and honour to your lower reproductive organs**: build a verbal relationship with your vulva and vagina and, as you do this, stroke and caress the vulva. This may sound silly, but words have power, and the vagina has a direct neurological connection to the brain. You can even write a letter to your vulva and vagina, if you find that easier. It will help to counter the effect of any negative and degrading words that you may have experienced or internalized about this part of the body. Do this when you are self-examining, or in bed when you get up in the morning or go to sleep.

* **Practise regular masturbation**: not only do many women find this embarrassing but, given how preoccupied and stressed we are with so many responsibilities in our lives, masturbation is often the last thing women are in the mood for or have time for. Yet it's such an empowering part of a loving relationship with yourself, enabling you

to explore your own needs, without the need for someone else to do that. Masturbation also has a range of proven health benefits, as well as improving sexual pleasure and increasing your chances of an orgasm. Learn to prioritize this as a regular part of your self-care.

❋   **Discuss and chat about vaginas and sex with your close girlfriends**: you'd be amazed how many women desperately need the permission that comes when someone else opens up on this topic, or about sexual pleasure. When we do this with people we trust, it can help us to feel secure and safe, and allows us to realize how many women have the same hang-ups, but feel isolated and alone about them. It can immediately put our minds at ease, or help to alert us to something that may need further input and support.

Introduction to your 12-week Conception Plan

This section gives you ideas for putting The Conception Plan's pillars into practice. The twelve weeks are divided into a week's preparation, five themed two-week periods of deep work, then a week of reflection.

As a lot of the stress in our lives comes from pushing ourselves beyond what our minds and bodies can bear at any one time, please don't see this as a must-do list, but rather as a rough guide that can be adapted. You don't have to do every single thing that is suggested, especially if your existing lifestyle is pretty different from what's suggested in the pillars. It may take time to cultivate new practices and behaviours, compared to what you're used to, so have patience with yourself.

Switching to a fertility-friendly lifestyle may feel difficult and you may feel resistance to some of the changes. Hopefully, having read the first part of this book, you'll understand the purpose of each of them, and that will help you. The places we hold the most resistance are often also the places where we stand to experience the greatest amount of growth. And looking at underlying emotions and trauma doesn't come easily to anybody. By giving yourself the time and space to spread out the changes over twelve weeks, taking small but powerful steps towards your goals, you will build confidence in yourself and your ability to become pregnant and will be able to support yourself in your pregnancy.

Week 1: new beginnings

*I love and trust my body; I cultivate patience and
compassion for its own timing.*

This is the preparation week, when you'll work out what will fit into
your life and will get started on some of the key changes.

First, the practical stuff

* Do you need to book a doctor's appointment? Do so if
  you've been trying for more than a year (aged thirty-five
  and under) or six months (over thirty-five, or have existing
  issues that may impact on fertility). And if you're worried
  about any gynaecological symptoms or conditions that may
  be having an impact on your ability to conceive. Your GP
  can run some basic tests to investigate.

* Consider getting tested for STDs. Infections can impact on
  the Fallopian tubes and/or create a suboptimal environment
  for implantation. This is true even for old infections that you
  may not be aware of having had.

* Is your cervical smear test up to date? If you are nervous
  or find it painful, do tell the nurse or doctor. They can use a
  smaller speculum and there are different positions that may
  help too. You can also bring a friend or someone you trust,
  for support. It's important to get this done if you're due,
  before you get started on trying to conceive.

* Are you taking a prenatal supplement (see page 89 for a
  guide to essential vitamins). This will not replace a nutritious
  diet, but it's important, both now and during pregnancy. Key
  nutrients that it should contain are folate, vitamin D, vitamin
  C, magnesium and zinc, but there are also others described
  in Chapter 6.

A NOTE ON THERAPY

The 12-week plan contains practices that will help you look into your emotions, understand yourself and become empowered to develop strategies. This can be emotionally painful and intense, as it may involve bringing up old trauma. TCP is not a substitute for therapy. Processing and integrating deep trauma – and especially trauma related to very intimate aspects of yourself – can require the help of an experienced therapist. Some of this therapy may be mind–body (somatic)-based, as well as traditional talking therapy.

Your conception journal

Your journal is going to have many important roles in this whole process. First, it's the place to let out all your fears, dark thoughts and middle-of-the-night worries, but also your hopes, dreams and gratitude. It's where you'll start to develop an intimate relationship with yourself. There's a kind of magic that happens when you write down all the confusing, conflicting, emotional maelstrom that may exist in your head. It can help release a lot of emotional charge stuck in the body and the nervous system, helping you to recognize stress that may have accumulated and emotional experiences that may not have been integrated. It will also help identify emotions that may not be your own.

Your journaling practice will also help to cultivate a sense of awareness around your own needs that will assist in establishing connections between the frontal part of the brain, which relates to concentration and decision-making, and the amygdala, which is related with emotional processing. It then becomes possible to deal with emotions with a sense of conscious perspective, where you're able to witness your pain, hold compassion for yourselves and create change.

How you can use your journal

❋ **Write for fifteen minutes every day**: write about what you feel like each day. You can use the specific journaling prompts and exercises that I suggest for each week or you can free-write. One good place to start is by writing about why you want to be a parent and how you think TCP will help.

❋ **Daily moment of gratitude**: wrap up your journaling each day by writing at least three things for which you are grateful. Expressing gratitude is powerful; doing it daily has been shown to protect you from stress and depression and make you see life from a more positive perspective. Your list doesn't have to include big things: even the smallest examples, such as your pet's soft fur against your skin or the warmth of your bed, are great. In fact the smaller they are, sometimes the more presence is required to appreciate them. Also remember to honour yourself for any progress you've made with TCP.

❋ **Daily affirmations**: I've shared an affirmation for each week of the plan. You can write them in your journal and repeat them out loud throughout the day. Or try chanting them and see how that feels. Alternatively, you can write them on sticky notes and put them up on your walls.

❋ **Consider writing about your dreams first thing when you get up**, otherwise you'll forget. Try not to be judgemental over their content or over-analytical: this is about expressing the subconscious, which can sometimes offer you downloads or messages that you would otherwise have been too distracted to notice.

Your journaling prompts

Do a feelings check-in (do this each day for the full twelve weeks) and notice how you are feeling right now.

- Where can you feel emotion in your body?
- What does it feel like? Can you describe it in words? Does it have a colour? Is it hot or cold?
- What is the emotion related to? Is it an emotion you recognize from the past or is it new?
- What triggered it?
- What lies beyond this emotion and trigger? Ask it, 'Do you have a message for me?' Don't judge the response that comes; simply write whatever comes to mind first, as well as any insights.

The idea is to learn to become familiar with *feeling* your feelings, both while you're journaling and, as you become more practised, during the day too. Sometimes your feelings may be really uncomfortable, such as anger or rage, embarrassment or shame. Instead of judging yourself for being a bad person, or trying to ignore or escape from your feelings, become curious about why a situation or person made you react in this way.

Daily meditation

Each week or fortnight there will be suggestions for meditations and/or visualizations for you to do, including a chakra activation. There is one activation for each of the seven chakras, spread out over the twelve weeks. Chakras are your emotional centres, and certain emotions are commonly related to specific chakras, where they can become embedded. Movement, breathwork, visualizations and tapping are ways in which you can process and clear any energetic densities that build up from unprocessed emotions during journaling. Try to do some meditation each day. Decide what time of day is best for you; you may find that after journaling or before bedtime is best. Start by doing just five minutes each day, but in time you can progress to much longer.

Third-eye chakra activation

The third-eye or brow chakra is connected to your sense of perception and thought-processing. It's also associated with the main endocrine organs in the brain, the hypothalamus and pituitary gland, which, as we saw earlier in the book, are very important when it comes to controlling reproduction. Clearing and activating this chakra at the beginning of the plan will reset your thoughts and give you mental clarity.

* Find a quiet space where you won't be disturbed.

* Close your eyes and take a couple of deep breaths in and out, focusing on your breath and drawing attention to your brow area. Continue to breathe deeply.

* Imagine a disc in the middle of your brow, then a violet light filtering in as you breathe in. Imagine the violet light getting brighter and larger and expanding your whole field of vision. Now imagine the disc spinning clockwise as you do this.

* Let the light expand with each breath and wash away any blockages.

* Allow your whole aura to be saturated with the colour violet.

* When you have done this for five minutes, open your eyes and go back to normal breathing.

If you wish, you can place a crystal on your brow or close to you. The ones that work best with this chakra are amethyst, fluorite and labradorite, all of which help connect you to your intuition, enhance spiritual awareness and promote mental clarity.

Daily visualization

See yourself as already a parent. Do this each day for five minutes for the full twelve weeks.

Imagine that you are (or your partner is) pregnant. Make a connection to your heart when you do this (you can place your hands over your heart to help). How does your life feel and look? What is your life like? How do *you* feel? What sort of parent are you? What are you doing differently compared to before? How do you speak to yourself? How do you treat yourself? What choices have you made that are different from before?

Starting off with the basics

You're going to begin with some of the fundamental changes that will make the biggest difference.

*   **Keep well hydrated and eat plenty of water-rich fruit and vegetables too**: this is key to supporting natural detoxification processes in the body and creating fertile cervical fluid. Plan how you'll do this; will you carry a water bottle with you?

*   **Cook one more meal than you would usually do, from scratch**: this is so much better than eating ready-made processed foods or takeaways, because you know the ingredients. If you are short of time, batch-cooking will be your friend here: can you cook once and eat twice or even three times? Over the twelve weeks, try to add another meal each week.

*   **Shop mindfully**: how can you plan to buy more local, seasonal and organic food? Is there a market near you? Or an organic shop?

*   **Plan a date night**: human connection — empathizing, listening and sharing — helps us tolerate and deal with stress. As well as doing this with your partner, plan

to see the closest people within your family and friends too.

* **Plan to have at least seven to nine hours of sleep each night**: this will reduce stress, help you eat better food and clear excess hormones, such as cortisol and oestrogen, from the body. What time do you need to go to bed in order to achieve this?

TCP self-care ideas: start the habit of looking after yourself

Begin the 12-week plan by doing the things that are good for you and that make you feel better. You don't have to do them all; and you can choose to do something else that works for you and fits the ethos of TCP.

* **Set aside a little time each day to do things that bring you pleasure,** whether that's having a bath and listening to your favourite podcast, treating yourself to a new book, gardening or spending time in nature, calling a good friend or listening to your favourite music.

* **Take an Epsom-salts bath**: add two cups of salts and soak for thirty minutes or more, helping you to absorb calming magnesium through the skin.

* **Practise earthing or grounding,** which means walking barefoot in your home and outside on grass. Doing this outside not only gives you the benefits of exercise and nature, but also helps to realign your biofield.

* **Consider booking a regular massage or seeing an osteopath or chiropractor** to help relieve tension and put your body and mind into a more relaxed state.

Cycle monitoring: three ways to start tracking your cycle

Cycle monitoring is a great way to learn about your body and respect your monthly variations and needs. As you get to know them over the course of the twelve weeks you can begin to treat them not as problems, but as the result of a beautifully orchestrated symphony of hormones providing clues as to what your body needs.

1. **Track your personal discharge**, and how it changes in response to the dynamic hormones over the course of your menstrual cycle. You might find the idea offputting, but vaginal discharge is one of the most important indicators of fertility, as well as being how your vagina naturally cleanses and protects itself from infection. Women often worry that their discharge is abnormal, because they're not familiar with what is normal. There will be slight variations in discharge between women, which is why it's important to get to know what is normal for you.

   * After menstruation (usually on Days 6–7 if you have a 28-day cycle) most women typically have no discharge or very little.

   * Roughly six days before ovulation (usually Days 8–14) you start producing and secreting more mucus. It starts as white/cream in colour and, as ovulation approaches, becomes slippery, wet and transparent.

   * The day before and the day of ovulation are peak time for the most fertile mucus, which looks and feels like egg white and helps sperm along. Ideally, you'll have sex each day during the time you have this discharge.

   * The luteal phase: after ovulation, when oestrogen declines and progesterone rises, discharge becomes sticky and thick and lacks elasticity. Women often notice it at this point: it can be quite dense and have a characteristic smell. This sort of mucus blocks the

passage of sperm, but the rise in progesterone helps with implantation.

* A number of factors can alter this process or lead to changes in mucus. Hormonal contraception stops cyclical variation in discharge, because it also blunts the variation in the underlying hormones. Pregnancy, menopause, vaginal infections, lubricants and drugs such as antihistamines can also affect the mucus.

2. **Monitor your basal body temperature**: there's a slight rise in temperature of 0.6–0.8 degrees that occurs just after ovulation, as progesterone rises. In pregnancy the temperature stays elevated and doesn't return to normal, as the level of progesterone remains consistently high. By the time the temperature rise reaches its peak, ovulation has already occurred – which means that it can't tell you about ovulation in advance. You need to make sure you've had at least five hours of sleep, that you take your temperature first thing in the morning and at the same time each day. For those who have a regular menstrual cycle, by charting your temperature over a few months, you can build a predictable pattern for the earliest and the latest that ovulation occurs for you. This can change: ovulation is sensitive to many factors, including stress. Instead of charting, you can also use a temperature device attached to an app. Or use an ovulation-predictor kit, where peeing on a stick detects the rise in luteinizing hormone (LH) that happens twenty-four to forty-eight hours before ovulation. However, these may not be reliable in women with PCOS (who have multiple surges of LH) or older women (whose LH can be higher).

3. **Monitor your other physical symptoms throughout the month, as well as your mood**: around ovulation, for example, you might feel mittelschmerz: a pain in the pelvis when a follicle swells and bursts to release the egg; or increased sex drive; breast sensitivity; an increased sense of

perception; sometimes mid-cycle bleeding; slight bloating; and an increased sense of well-being (see page 158).

Planning

At the beginning of each week get into the habit of planning how you're going to look after yourself according to each of the five pillars. Ask yourself, 'What would feel good to do for my body this week?'

Your plan can be as detailed or as simple as you like. The key is to write it down in your journal. Writing it down will focus your mind and make it more likely to happen. For example, for your exercise plan you might write: five x 10-minute yoga every morning, two x 30-minute Pilates classes Mondays and Thursdays or thirty minutes of brisk walking daily. Some people, especially those who are busy, like to plan the sex too (you may not). Aim for two to three times a week, all month as well as in the fertile period, but remember: none of this should feel like a chore and, if it does, stop and assess why you're meeting resistance.

Weeks 2 and 3: clean and clear

*I honour the different phases of my reproductive cycle
and the blessings and growth each one brings.*

The theme of this fortnight is about clearing away whatever is not helping you. That might be in a practical sense – as in replacing products that contain reprotoxins or foods that aren't helpful for fertility – and emotionally. You'll practise paying attention to your thoughts and ruminations, seeing them for what they are: just thoughts; and replacing them with those that are healthier, when they aren't serving you.

Your conception journal

Your journaling prompts

✳ When were the times in your life when you felt you couldn't fully express yourself or step into your power? Perhaps you felt you had to conform or not upset someone?

* How do you feel about your role in life? Are there aspects you resent and, if so, why?

* Do you have any difficulty accepting yourself?

* Do you hold on to grudges and find it hard to confront people over being treated badly?

* What have your relationships been like, and how have they made you feel?

* Do you have any unexpressed anger? What is it, and where in your body are you storing it?

* Do you have fears or misgivings about becoming a mother or father? If so, where did they come from? Read the section on the Mother Wound (Chapter 5) and see if it rings true.

Journaling exercise: write a letter

Think of a difficult relationship in your present or past and write that person a letter. You don't need to give them the letter, so you can write exactly what you feel. The idea is to learn to express your emotions. If, after doing this, you realize that some of your reactions in the present are being triggered by the past, write this down too. By exploring the hidden meaning behind present reactions you can start to address the root causes. Sometimes burning the letter is helpful, in a small ceremony (do it over the sink or put it onto a log fire!). You can repeat this exercise over the twelve weeks if you wish, for different people.

Daily meditation

Solar-plexus chakra activation

This meditation will help to connect you with your inner source of power, enabling you to create change, as well as identifying any areas where you may be feeling disempowered. Crystals you can use include amber, tiger's eye, pyrite, sunstone and golden topaz.

* Close your eyes and imagine a ball of yellow in your midriff. Feel it heat up into a ball of fire.

* Place your hands on this area and breathe deeply into it, allowing any emotions of anger, control, frustration, fear, judgement and limitation to rise to the surface.

* Visualize a yellow/orange flame moving through and out of your body, then observe these feelings dissolving, while releasing all tension and fear.

* Now say out loud the following affirmations:

  o I stand in my personal power.

  o I feel motivated and confident to pursue my dreams.

  o I honour the innate power within me.

  o I am strong and can create positive change in my life.

  o I am ready for something better.

* Open your eyes and bring your attention back to your surroundings.

A mindful-thought detox

Notice how you speak to yourself during the day. When negative thoughts come towards you – for example, 'I'm a failure' or 'I'm not enough' – see if you can become a passive observer of them, as if they were clouds drifting across a landscape, without attaching emotion to them. Understand that your thoughts don't define you. They're simply outputs of your consciousness.

You can also write them down and really look at what they are saying. Ask yourself, 'Is this thought really true?' What's the narrative you've fed yourself about why you've reached that conclusion? Recognize that most of these narratives have fear at their root. What if you changed your perspective and viewed them through a different lens of compassion and forgiveness? Would you feel differently about yourself? Try empowering affirmations that encourage new neural connections, such as this one: 'I am fully embodied, I am loved, I am present, I am enough, I am a magnet for life and abundance to flow through me, I am preparing my mind, body and spirit for the great miracles coming my way.'

Cycle monitoring: noticing any abnormalities

By the end of this fortnight you'll be three weeks into your cycle monitoring – and you may find you're not following the exact course of a regular 28-day cycle.

Understanding the normal changes that take place in a menstrual cycle is important, although every woman can have variations in her cycle from time to time. However, if any of the features below keep recurring, it's important to raise them with your doctor.

* **Signs of ovulation before Day 14, such as a temperature spike and/or fertile mucus**: with age, the first or follicular phase of the cycle (from Day 1 until ovulation) can start to become irregular or shorten. This means that ovulation and the fertile window shifts earlier too.

* **Basal body temperature that's slow to rise, or there's a smaller rise than normal (less than 0.2°C)**: this can indicate a luteal-phase deficiency (linked to lower progesterone).

* **Absent spikes of temperature and/or non-conducive cervical mucus**: this may indicate that you haven't ovulated this month.

* **A follicular phase that's less than ten days (that is, ovulation occurs before Day 10)**: this may mean the uterine lining does not have time to thicken enough for implantation.

* **A follicular phase lasting longer than twenty days (that is, ovulation occurring after Day 20)**: the resulting slow rise in oestrogen may lead to lower egg quality.

✳ **A luteal phase that lasts ten days or less, or your period arrives ten days or less after ovulating**: this can indicate a luteal phase defect that reflects low progesterone levels that may not be enough for implantation.

✳ **Bleeding or spotting between periods (intermenstrual bleeding)**, although this may be normal and can be due to ovulation, but may also indicate a luteal phase defect.

✳ **Heavy menstrual bleeding (HMB or menorrhagia)**: this is defined as bleeding that exceeds 80ml or that lasts for longer than seven days. If you often flood through clothes, notice large clots, have to change protection every hour, double up on your protection or arrange your life around your period, that is likely to be HMB.

✳ **Painful periods**: if your periods stop you from being able to do normal activities, or you find yourself taking a variety of painkillers to manage.

✳ **Bleeding after sex.**

A focus on toxin-free living

For these two weeks, focus on ways to detoxify your lifestyle. Here are some ideas to start with, or look back at Chapter 9.

✳ **Go natural**: each time you use up a cleaning or beauty product, keep replacing it with a more natural version.

✳ **Do a plastic detox**: can you buy more of your food ingredients without plastic? Switch to loose fruit and vegetables, rather than bagged. Find your local refill shop for dry ingredients (some health-food shops do this too). Switch from a plastic water bottle to a metal or glass one. Store food in the fridge in ceramic or glass rather than plastic. Don't heat food in plastic containers. When you buy food, take your own (metal or glass) containers.

✳ **Go unscented, or make sure only natural scents are used**: most scents are synthetic, so they are worth avoiding. Products to check include washing powder, washing-up liquid and other cleaning products, perfume, deodorants, face and body moisturizer, make-up, shampoo and conditioner, air fresheners and scented candles.

Seven ways to support your body's detox functions

The main ways in which you detox chemicals are via the liver, by elimination through the gut and via the skin. You should already be drinking enough water (between two and three litres a day), which helps. But also:

1. Reduce your consumption of coffee to one cup a day (or two of tea).

2. Stop smoking, if you do smoke.

3. Keep your alcohol intake minimal (ideally zero), as it can lead to inflammation and create hormonal imbalances.

4. Treat constipation through diet and exercise, if you suffer from this. Toxins can be reabsorbed from the stool via a constipated lower colon, which sits next to the ovaries and uterus.

5. Consume more fibre in your diet by adding vegetables and good carbs (see page 85). This will help keep your bowel habit regular — you're aiming for once or twice a day.

6. Plan your meals with plenty of vegetables: raw, steamed and seasonal (see page 80).

7. Add in regular daily movement: all kinds of exercise counts!

Detox your sleep habits

Focusing on getting better sleep can be a game-changer for stress levels and hormones.

* **Get ten to twenty minutes of daylight each morning** – ideally sunlight first thing. Light in your eyes gets your body clock into sync and eventually stimulates the evening release of the sleep hormone melatonin (which has a knock-on effect on mood-boosting serotonin too).

* **Turn off screens and turn down the lights at least one hour before bed** – and ideally two hours.

* **Have sex** – it boosts the hormones oxytocin and prolactin while reducing cortisol, all of which help to promote sleep.

* **Take vitamin D daily** – low levels of this vitamin are associated with sleepiness, reduced sleep duration and increased interruptions during sleep.

* **Create rituals around bedtime** to help get you in the mood for sleep, whether it's having a soothing candlelit bath or gently massaging your face as you cleanse.

* **Take a magnesium supplement at night** or add Epsom salts to your bath before bedtime; both of these help to relax the muscles.

* **Some botanicals,** such as lavender and lemon balm, may help with bedtime stress and anxiety.

* **Eat foods rich in tryptophan,** such as free-range turkey, fish, cheese, pumpkin and sesame seeds, as well as foods rich in magnesium, such as avocados, cashews, Brazil nuts and dark chocolate, all of which can help boost mood, relaxation and improve sleep.

* **Eat pistachios before bedtime;** they contain natural melatonin, which will help you drift off.

Weeks 4 and 5: getting in tune with your body and emotions

*My mind, body and spirit are harmonizing
together in the best possible way to help me to have a baby.*

This fortnight you'll be practising tuning into your body's needs and trusting that it's going to tell you what it needs: does it require more activity or rest? Massage or sleep? Changing your exercise and eating according to your menstrual cycles is key, as is tuning into your inner guidance. It's time to commit to being more attentive to you.

Your conception journal

Now that you've been practising the feelings check-in for a few weeks you may have noticed that being more aware can sometimes intensify your symptoms, creating discomfort and resistance. If you need it, ask for help or support, whether that's from a professional or from a loved one. But you may also have noticed that you were able to hold yourself with compassion and patience while experiencing any difficult emotions.

Your journaling prompts

* What is currently making you feel overwhelmed?

* Are you trying to control all the circumstances around your infertility?

* Are any of your personal boundaries being challenged or disrespected? How can you hold them better?

* Are you living with too much external stimulation? If so, what can you scale back?

* Are you lacking connection with other people? Do you feel lonely and disconnected? If so, who can you reach out to?

❉ Do you find yourself ruminating too much over the past? Or worrying too much about the future? What helps you stay in the present?

❉ Are you looking after yourself and your own needs? How can you do this?

❉ Are you being compassionate towards yourself? How can you be kinder to yourself?

❉ Do you have enough emotional support to call on in your life? Can you ask for more?

❉ When your emotions are triggered, do you give yourself the space and time to deal with this? How and when will you do this from now on?

Daily meditation

Crown-chakra activation

This will help you to step into a different stream of consciousness where all possibilities exist, and to connect with spirit. Crystals that you can use include clear quartz, selenite, white agate, apophyllite and diamonds.

❉ Sit in a quiet place, resting your palms facing upwards in your lap, and breathe deeply, taking your breath all the way down your spine and back up.

❉ Straighten your spine and lift your head, so that the crown of your head is pointed upwards.

❉ Close your eyes and roll them slightly upwards.

❉ Place the tip of your tongue on the roof of your mouth.

❉ Visualize a bright white light at the top of your head, glowing and streaming through your body and out into your aura.

* As the light spirals through you, say out loud the following affirmations:

    o I am safe, nourished and protected.

    o The intelligence of something far bigger and more infinite flows through me.

    o Everything in my life is unfolding as it should and is connecting me to my deepest purpose.

    o I trust in the divine order and flow.

* Imagine every cell of your body soaking up this light. Allow it to flow through your core and feel it activating you.

* Open your eyes and bring your attention back to your surroundings.

Cycle monitoring: exercise in tune with your menstrual cycle

The hormonal changes that take place during the menstrual cycle can affect sleep, appetite, stress, how energetic we feel and how much pain is experienced. Adjusting your exercise according to your menstrual cycle is a great way to respect your body's natural needs and optimize the benefits of exercise.

When you lean into the phase that your body is currently experiencing, you're also helping to support your hormonal health and balance. This is a guide to how your body may feel in the different phases of your cycle.

Follicular phase

As oestrogen levels rise, you'll feel more energetic. The central nervous system forms new connections more easily right now, so this is a great time to try novel forms of exercise and sport. This is the best time to do higher-intensity exercise (although don't go too hard – see the guidelines in Chapter 7), such as running, dancing, dynamic yoga or strength training with heavier weights.

During ovulation

Oestrogen levels increase further and you reach your apex of energy at this point, so you can keep working out as in the follicular phase. Group sport or dancing is good, because at this time in the cycle your body craves connection with others. However, if you experience pain or bloating during ovulation, you may want to switch to the guidelines given below during menstruation.

Luteal phase

Oestrogen levels decline, and progesterone rises, leading to fatigue and a decline in endurance. You naturally become more inward-focused and start to retain more water. The increased body temperature in this phase can also mean that cardiovascular exercise isn't as well tolerated and the time to exhaustion is shorter. You may find it more comfortable and beneficial to do lower-impact sport, such as Pilates, walking, yoga or swimming.

Just before and during menstruation

Many women avoid exercise during menstruation. You might have less stamina, some bloating or cramping as well as headaches, which can all make you less likely to want to move. If your bleeding is heavy or you suffer from painful periods, it may be best to rest. However, exercise hydrates the fascia that surrounds different organs and can help to relieve tension and cramps, so you may find that gentle exercise makes you feel a lot better. Try slow, meditative yoga or stretching. If you want to do a little more, try Pilates and sculpting with light weights. Walking outside is good for everyone: early daylight and spending time in nature will regulate your hypothalamus, which in turn will regulate your stress response and endocrine system.

Breathwork: deepening the connection with yourself

Add intentional breathing into your daily practice. It doesn't need to be complicated, and it only takes five minutes (or even less). You can do it in the morning and/or whenever you feel you need to calm your nervous system. Breathwork helps to activate the vagus nerve, which tells your nervous system that you are safe, reduces stress hormones and improves a measure of stress called heart-rate variability. Repeat one of these exercises five to ten times first thing in the morning, and however many times you need to during the day.

* **Paced respiration**: this is where your out-breath is longer than your in-breath. So, for example, breathe out for a count of five and in for three; or out for six and in for four.

* **Box breathing**: with one hand on your tummy and the other on your chest, feel the expansion and release – inhale through the nose for four counts, hold for four, then exhale for four and hold for four.

Weeks 6 and 7: nourish and nurture

I love and honour my womb space and
my body as a portal of new life coming through me.

Congratulations: you've now done five weeks of great work on yourself. During this two-week period you're going to focus on food as your nutritional powerhouse, packed with everything you need to optimize your fertility. But this is also a time to focus on nurturing yourself and further unpack your relationship with yourself. Doing TCP, you are already honouring your body and your mind, because you have committed to keeping regular promises about things you will do to look after yourself.

Your conception journal

Your journaling prompts

* When in your life were you prevented from being able to express and explore yourself in the creative or sexual sphere?

* How did you deal with authority figures in your life? Did you find yourself giving way to their needs, even if it meant compromising your own needs and boundaries?

* Have you previously felt invaded or suppressed, and has this left you with feelings of rage and anger?

* Do you hold on to any guilt and/or shame from previous experiences?

* Has there been significant conflict between you and your parents?

* Do you find yourself holding on to old wounds and lashing out in the most unexpected circumstances?

* Have you been allowed to use and cultivate your gifts and talents?

* Do you find yourself pushing people away, for fear they may get too close?

* Do you doubt whether you're enough, as you are?

* Though you want to be a mother (or father), do you have doubts about whether you will be a good one or about the sort of mother (or father) you'll be?

Journaling exercise: 'Dear me'

Write a letter to yourself, giving yourself permission to experience all the feelings that are normally stigmatized, such as shame, anger, embarrassment and loneliness. Instead of judging yourself, see your emotions as what they are: a natural consequence of having experienced trauma. Write to yourself as if you were your best friend, letting go of judgement and using words that are soothing and understanding. When you've finished, read the letter again and soak in the words.

Daily meditation

Sacral-chakra activation

Activating this centre helps us to connect to our inner source of creativity and sexuality. It also helps to restore balance in our relationships. Crystals that you can use include carnelian, jasper and citrine.

* Sit or lie down with the soles of your feet touching and your knees open.

* Close your eyes and take deep breaths in and out, up and down your spine.

* Visualize an orange ball of light in your womb space and spreading out into your body and into your aura. You need to include the aura (or the biofield, if you prefer) as well as the body, for the reasons mentioned earlier (see page 39).

* Say the following affirmations out loud:

  o I am a sexual being who is deserving of pleasure.

  o Creation flows through me with ease and grace.

  o I celebrate the flow of life within me.

  o I am free to express my sensuality.

* Open your eyes and bring your attention back to your surroundings.

Focus on food

As we've discussed, there are so many reasons to eat well. The right food creates the right epigenetic environment for all your cells, including the sperm and egg. It keeps you in an anti-inflammatory state, which is pro-fertility. It supplies the body not only with the ingredients that make the sperm and the egg, but also with those of the body's fertility support system: hormones, neurotransmitters and immune chemicals. And as well as affecting the body, food also affects the brain, including the hippo-campus, which controls stress, which in turn has an indirect effect on fertility.

How will you fill your plate?

Here are a few ideas to focus on during this fortnight, but refer back to Chapter 6 for more.

* **Vegetables of all colours**: think rainbow, raw, steamed, seasonal and fermented.

* **Plenty of quality protein**: grass-fed organic meat and poultry, organic/wild fish, seafood and especially plant protein, such as buckwheat, brown rice, lentils, chickpeas, mung beans, quinoa, nut butters and seeds.

* **Good fats**: cold-pressed nut and seed oils and olive oil, oily fish, nuts and seeds, avocado, ghee and coconut oil.

* **Low-GI carbs**: quinoa, spelt, bulgur wheat and brown rice, as well as parsnips, sweet potatoes, beetroot, carrots and other root vegetables.

* **Grass-fed dairy products**: or non-dairy alternatives.

Maximize nutrition and absorption

* **Add probiotic foods.** These contain good bacteria that allow the beneficial bacteria in our guts to proliferate. They include fermented foods such as kefir, kombucha, sauerkraut and apple cider vinegar.

* **Eat prebiotics.** The fibre in these foods acts as food for the microbiome. Prebiotics include apples, bananas, flaxseeds, chia seeds, garlic, onions, leeks and asparagus.

* **Chewing well** breaks down food so it can be digested better. It also helps your brain and digestive system to

relax, so that food moves more smoothly through the digestive tract.

* **Smell your food before eating.** This helps start the process of secreting the enzymes required to digest food.

* **Adding (gentle) spices** such as ginger, cumin and black pepper speeds up nutrient absorption.

* **Have plenty of warming drinks throughout the day** (ideally caffeine- and all sugar-free!) to help your body to metabolize food. But don't drink while you're eating, as it can dilute stomach acid.

* **To help digestion, have a tablespoon of apple cider vinegar or a squeeze of lemon in a glass of water before you eat.**

* **Make a smoothie.** This is a great way to eat more raw foods. When you blend fruit and vegetables it breaks down the fibre so you can absorb the nutrients more easily. Just make sure it's more vegetable than fruit.

Top-ten fertility foods

These foods have been chosen because they contain plenty of phyto-chemicals and other helpful nutrients; you don't have to fixate on eating them, but they are good to keep in mind as you focus on food this fortnight.

1. **Salmon** is a low-mercury fish, a good source of protein, rich in Omega 3 and vitamin D as well as selenium. Buy organic/wild whenever possible, and eat up to three portions a week.

2. **Berries** contain all the antioxidant benefits of red and purple phytonutrients as well as fibre, plus they are low-GI.

3. **Quinoa** is a low-GI carb that's also a great source of plant protein, as well as zinc and folate.

4. **Lentils** are a good source of plant-based protein, plus folate and iron.

5. **Cruciferous vegetables**, such as broccoli, cabbage, watercress and kale, are key in helping your liver to detox used-up oestrogen, which helps to keep your hormones in balance.

6. **Eggs** contain choline, which studies suggest is key in reducing the risk of birth defects. They also contain iron, calcium, zinc, Omega 3, vitamin D and a range of B vitamins. *Note*: avoid eating raw eggs, due to the small risk of salmonella food poisoning.

7. **Flaxseeds** are rich in Omega 3, B vitamins, manganese and magnesium, and are also a source of phytoestrogens that diminish the action of the synthetic xenoestrogens found in the environment (see Chapter 9).

8. **Avocados** are an important source of Omega 3 and other good fats, contain plenty of fibre and support your liver to detox used-up hormones.

9. **Turmeric** is a potent anti-inflammatory agent and helps to lower stress hormones.

10. **Cinnamon** has antibacterial properties and can also help keep blood sugar balanced.

Cycle monitoring: eat in tune with your cycle

Follicular phase

This is the stage of your cycle when your body is best at digesting raw food, so keep cooking minimal, in order to preserve the nutrient content. Eat more vegetables, lean protein, beans and nuts.

As follicles grow and the endometrial lining renews, protein is especially important. Make sure yours is predominantly from fish or plant sources. Foods containing good Omega 3:Omega 6 ratios, such as avocados, eggs and salmon, as well as full-fat grass-fed organic dairy products, are beneficial. Vitamin E can help to support the developing eggs, so include wholegrains, sweet potatoes and cold-pressed unrefined oils.

Around ovulation

Boost vitamin B levels to promote ovulation by eating leafy greens, organic meat and wholegrains. As oestrogen reaches a peak, incorporate lots of vegetables and fruit for their antioxidant benefits, and lots of fibre to ensure that excess oestrogen is being metabolized. Zinc helps with cell division and progesterone production, so eat eggs, wholegrains, oysters and crab.

Luteal phase

Your digestion will benefit from support now, so eat warming foods such as stews, soups, broths and curries. Increase your natural progesterone levels by eating foods that promote progesterone production, such as cabbage, kale, broccoli, Brussels sprouts, spinach, wholegrains, pumpkin seeds, nuts, bananas and shellfish. These will also support the liver in eliminating waste hormones and will help to counteract any excess oestrogen. Though you may be craving it, limit processed food, refined sugar and caffeine and replace them with low-glycaemic-load carbs, such as sweet potatoes, wholegrains, dried fruit and berries. This will help reduce mood swings. This is also the best time to eat pineapple, which contains bromelain that may help implantation of the embryo.

Just before and during menstruation

Rather than eating food that is raw, this is the time to focus on cooking and eating stews and soups as well as roasted vegetables. Eat more iron-rich foods, such as beetroot and organic meat, as well as seaweed and seafood, leafy greens, dried fruit and nuts and seeds. Include foods rich in vitamin C to help with iron absorption, such as citrus fruit, mangoes, tomatoes, peas and watercress.

Avocados and cruciferous vegetables help the liver to process excess oestrogen. And upping your fibre content with wholegrains, chia seeds, beans, brown rice and, of course, vegetables and fruit helps to move excess hormones out of the body.

Reduce refined sugar, artificial sweeteners and simple carbs, which disturb insulin regulation and increase inflammatory chemicals (prostaglandins and prostacyclins) that can make periods heavier and more painful and may drive PMS. Substitute with coconut sugar and dates.

Eliminate trans fats, as they increase inflammation and insert themselves into cell membranes, which can cause cell dysfunction and interfere with cell signalling. Increase healthy fats and Omega 3 (hemp seed, coconut, chia seed, flaxseed, grass-fed ghee, cold-pressed olive, evening-primrose and sea-buckthorn oils).

Support your liver function (also key for getting rid of used hormones) by eating these foods: beetroot, artichokes and dandelion leaf.

Reduce alcohol and caffeine, as they are inflammatory.

Including natural probiotics, such as sauerkraut, kefir or kombucha, in your diet can help your gut produce the neurotransmitters that your brain needs to regulate pain and help stabilize mood.

Brown spotting before a period may be a sign of low progesterone levels. So help boost progesterone levels by eating progesterone-building foods such as salmon, cruciferous vegetables and nuts.

Irregular bleeding is often an indicator of irregular ovulation. Addressing stress levels, and particularly keeping blood sugar even by avoiding refined sugar and sticking to high-GI carbs, can help improve the pattern of ovulation and bleeding.

NURTURE FROM NATURE

Spend time outdoors in nature as often as you can, to lower nervous-system arousal, enhance the immune system and improve mood. Researchers have found that being in nature reduces feelings of loneliness, promotes calm and lifts mood among patients. The healing benefits of nature are referred to as ecopsychology.

Revive with self-care

❉ **Move your body**: any kind of exercise is key for managing stress, because it increases the ability of nerve cells and tissue to regenerate (see page 102 for suggestions).

❉ **Take a class/learn something new**: women's oestrogen levels can be lower than optimal because of situations where they're forced into more extreme levels of independence, such as having to manage without enough support. Some ways of restoring normal oestrogen involve spending time with friends, feeling heard and listened to in a relationship, and becoming comfortable with the idea of depending on someone, who might be a teacher for something new in your life.

❉ **Play hard**: being playful with other people takes you out of survival mode and into a relaxed state.

❉ **Dance**: this is a brilliant way to express yourself; plus, it will improve your self-esteem as well as your cognitive function.

❉ **Art**: this can be a good way of expressing emotions that are difficult to articulate – something that children often do without realizing it. It can help you see some of your internal landscape more clearly.

❉ **Fake being stress-free**, and your body and brain may actually believe it! Standing in a power pose – hands on hips, head high and chest out – for just two minutes can increase testosterone by 20 per cent and reduce cortisol by 25 per cent.

Weeks 8 and 9: pleasure, love and sex

I nurture and recognize the creative power within me.

The focus this fortnight is on love: both love for yourself and love in significant relationships. This is a chance to take a deep dive into sexuality and libido, as well as communication and connection

Your conception journal

A reminder, as you continue doing the feelings check-in, that your emotions are helpful messages inviting you to unravel aspects of yourself. Keep allowing yourself full permission to feel your emotions, without judgement, noticing where in your body you feel them most intensely. And see if you can tap into the wisdom of what your body is wanting to tell you and what it needs. When emotions feel too strong or unfamiliar, you may notice that your nervous system shuts down and you feel numb as it tries to protect you. But as you are gradually becoming more familiar with being present in emotional intensity, you may notice that this happens less often.

Your journaling prompts

Read these questions each morning or evening and write down whatever comes up.

* Have you ever been made to feel shameful about being a woman or about your sexual desires?

* Do you feel anger and resentment over how you've been treated sexually in the past?

* Does having sexual needs and desires make you feel shame?

* Do you find it difficult to accept the concept of self-pleasure and self-love, and if so, why?

*   Have you faced situations where you've been rejected or abandoned?

*   Have you felt taken advantage of, and that others abused your good intentions?

*   What was your first sexual encounter like? And subsequent ones thereafter?

*   Do you feel that your boundaries have been kept and respected or dishonoured and disrespected? How did that leave you feeling?

*   Do you often feel disempowered? Do you find it hard to stand up for yourself? If yes, what prevents you from doing so?

Daily meditation

Root-chakra activation

Connecting with this centre will help you to tap into feeling safe, grounded and supported, as well as helping you to have faith. Crystals that you can use are haematite, smoky quartz, black tourmaline, shungite, red garnet, black onyx, rhodonite and ruby.

*   Either stand or sit with your feet on the ground. Close your eyes.

*   Bring your attention to the base of your spine and visualize a red ball of light there.

*   Breathe into the red light and allow it to expand into the lower part of your body, gradually rising and then extending out into your aura.

*   As you exhale, spiral the red light down your body and spine, all the way through your feet into the ground. As you inhale, send the red light up through your body. Repeat several times.

* Allow the light to move through and around you, bathing you in crimson.

* Chant the word 'Lammmmm' several times over a few minutes.

* After you have done this, say out loud:

  o I am grounded and centred.

  o I am deeply connected to the Earth.

  o I belong.

  o I am safe and provided for.

  o I trust all of my needs are being met.

  o I am enough and I have everything I need.

* Bring your awareness to your breath. Slowly open your eyes and bring your attention back to your surroundings.

Regular masturbation

Spend time getting to know what gives you pleasure. This may be the last thing you're in the mood for or think you can put aside time for, but exploring your own needs is key to a loving relationship with yourself and is hugely empowering too. It also has fertility benefits, relieving stress, improving sleep and increasing your chance of an orgasm when you are with a partner.

Sex to suit your menstrual cycle

The hormone fluctuations of your menstrual cycle don't only dictate the chances of conception, but also how sex can be optimized.

Follicular phase

Oestrogen, progesterone and testosterone start off low and rise towards ovulation. In order to increase hormone levels to maximize arousal and pleasure – oestrogen in particular – you will require longer fore-play and stimulation. Engaging in self-care and pleasure during the day (see Chapter 10) will improve your libido. Equally, your partner needs to be patient and understanding in allowing more time for arousal.

Around ovulation

Oestrogen and testosterone levels naturally rise, and you'll probably not require as long to become aroused. Most women crave more sex or sexual encounters at this time. This is also the ideal time when sex can be more experimental and energetic, so don't hold back!

Luteal phase

Although progesterone initially rises just after ovulation, it then begins to decline, as do testosterone and oestrogen. You may not be in the mood for sex, especially in the lead-up to your period. If you are, follow the principles of the follicular phase. This is a time when women may be more uncomfortable or experience pain during sex, especially premenstrually.

During menstruation

Many women abstain from sex now, but you don't have to. Some women find menstrual sex very enjoyable and/or that it releases tension and relieves pain, including headaches and menstrual cramps.

Focus on pleasure

The starting point for pleasure is cultivating a deeper sense of connection with yourself and with your partner.

* **Connect with your partner via touch**: massage can help relieve muscle tension and improve blood and energetic

flow, while releasing endorphins and reducing stress hormones.

✳ **Commit to regular acts of self-love**: that could be running a bath, doing a hobby you love or spending time in nature.

✳ **Don't underestimate the importance of foreplay,** and not just in the bedroom, but throughout the whole day. A dynamic process of flirtation should ideally unfold for many hours prior to actually being together and ready to have sex, because the anticipation is what is sexually arousing and increases the chance of orgasm.

✳ **Spend time gazing into each other's eyes**: eye contact has been shown to activate nerve projections that connect with the prefrontal cortex of the brain, which processes empathy and matches emotions. The long gaze is involved in mirror-neuron behaviour, coordinating thoughts, feelings and actions based on how we perceive others feel about us.

✳ **As well as focusing on the clitoris and sometimes the G-spot**, explore stimulation around the whole of the front vaginal wall and deeper tissue, because orgasm can come from stimulation here too.

Notes about libido for partners of women

✳ Words matter, when it comes to sex. The right words can neurobiologically prime a woman's sexual response. A message to partners: praise your partner, tell her how much you value her and how beautiful she is.

✳ Around the time of ovulation, women's heightened levels of testosterone generally mean more risk-taking and being drawn to more unpredictable, volatile men. But in the luteal phase, as testosterone declines, they may be drawn towards the comfort of more predictable behaviour and reliability. And so spicing things up appears to be a necessary part of the female biological condition around the time when she's most fertile.

*   From time to time do something spontaneous and unpredictable to induce the beneficial stress that is arousing to women. For some, this might be a trip away together; for others, it might be being adventurous in the bedroom.

*   Women who have lower baseline levels of oestrogen – such as those who are perimenopausal (in the time prior to menopause, when symptoms can be commonly experienced), in the menopause or experiencing more stress – need more non-sexual touch to raise oestrogen levels as well as more foreplay. Kissing, cuddling and verbal compliments can help.

*   According to Tibetan, Chinese and Tantric medicine, for a woman to feel she can surrender and soften during sex, her 'moon centres' need to be stimulated. This triggers the release of neurochemicals that diminish thought-processing and encourage disinhibition and surrender. They are found at the nape of the neck, cheeks, lips, forehead and hands. There are additional moon centres in erogenous zones, such as the breasts, earlobes, inside of the thighs, clitoris and anterior vagina, and one in the uterus that is stimulated indirectly.

*   Stroking a woman has a whole range of great effects: it regulates her nervous system, reduces blood pressure and increases oxytocin, leading to an increase in affection and trust. It also helps to deactivate the amygdala, the fear and anxiety centre of the brain, which is necessary for sexual arousal to occur.

Notes about libido for partners of men

＊ As men become more loving and invested in relationships, their testosterone levels go down. To give them passion-sustaining bursts of testosterone, they require regular communication and praise for their achievements, no matter how small.

＊ By making nurturing and loving comments during sex, men can learn to rewire their brains, so that they form a connection with the prefrontal cortex, which helps them to stay more present and to build deeper love during sex. Talking also helps women feel valued and safe during sex, when positive loving comments encourage their levels of oestrogen and oxytocin to surge and their love and connection to build.

＊ Desire grows when you're apart. Sleeping in separate bedrooms may seem counterintuitive, but when you're not constantly in the presence of someone else, it keeps your bioenergetic field more polarized. Then when you do come together for sex, not only will you have renewed lust for one another, but you'll likely have better and more powerful sex too.

Focus on relationships

Chronic stress not only exhausts both partners, eroding libido and the desire for sex, but also leads to very different responses in men and women. Generally speaking, I've seen that stress initiates a need for women to talk and connect, but for men to shut down and detach. And so the longer stress lasts, the longer it means that both partners are not getting their needs met. Aside from the measures already discussed when it comes to dealing with stress, what else can help?

✳ **Doing the meditations in this plan,** which will help to connect you back with your body. Meditation can help restore testosterone levels in men too.

✳ **Spending time outdoors**: natural light will boost libido, and being in nature will cut stress levels and help optimize hormone levels.

✳ **Learning to enforce healthy boundaries** that honour you and the people around you; and if someone attempts to breach this, become comfortable with saying no.

✳ **Cultivating clear communication with your partner and people you're close to,** feeling free to express your feelings and having a willingness to commit to loving and supporting one another.

Nutrition for pleasure

Plan some meals that include foods with the following libido-supporting effects. They are not the only foods you should eat, but should be incorporated into a balanced diet.

✳ **Foods with high levels of zinc** support testosterone levels. They include pumpkin seeds, beans, grass-fed beef, crab, lobster and oysters.

✳ **Foods high in the amino acid carnitine** (found in grass-fed organic meat, fish and wholegrains) are beneficial in optimizing blood flow to the reproductive organs.

✳ **Nuts and seeds** are rich in Omega 3 as well as the amino acid arginine, which can boost libido.

✳ **Beetroot** is very high in nitrates, which help to expand blood vessels and increase the chance of experiencing pleasure during intercourse. Other foods high in nitrates are spinach, rocket, lettuce, celery and radish.

✻ **Green tea** contains catechins, which increase nitric oxide, help to dilate blood vessels and increase blood flow to the pelvic organs (but be mindful of the caffeine in green tea).

✻ **Dark chocolate**, in moderation, can help to lead to the release of the happy hormone serotonin, plus a brain chemical called phenethylamine that has aphrodisiac and mood-lifting effects.

✻ **Fatty fish**, such as salmon and sardines, are a good source of Omega 3, which increases dopamine, the same chemical we get from being love-struck. It is also obtained from hemp seed, coconut, chia seed, flaxseed, grass-fed ghee, cold-pressed olive oil, evening-primrose and sea-buckthorn oils.

✻ **Fruit** contains flavonoids that can reduce blood pressure and therefore reduce the incidence of erectile dysfunction.

✻ **Fresh pomegranate**, without added sugar, helps to boost testosterone, antioxidants and blood flow.

✻ **Watermelon** is a source of vitamin B, which is important in managing stress and increases libido by helping to keep cortisol low.

Sexercise!

Regular exercise not only improves libido and blood flow to the reproductive organs, but makes you feel better about yourself. Try one (or more) of the following suggestions, which can improve sex too.

✻ **Kegel exercises** can help tone the pelvic floor, improving sexual pleasure and helping to reduce the chance of premature ejaculation.

✻ **Walking** has been shown to improve libido and reduce the risk of erectile dysfunction.

❋ **Consider exercising together**, because studies show that challenging physical activities spark arousal. Swimming builds endurance, boosts blood flow, reduces stress and improves flexibility, all of which can help improve sexual performance. Yoga can help to improve desire, arousal, orgasm and lubrication.

❋ **Real rest** is important too. Try to get seven to nine hours of sleep each night, because your circadian rhythms have a great effect on your libido.

Bedroom detox

We spend one-third of our lives in bed, so it's an important place to keep toxin-free.

❋ **Air the bedroom regularly**: this helps get rid of indoor air pollution as well as moisture that can build up and cause mould growth.

❋ **Minimize Wi-Fi exposure** by keeping your phone out of the bedroom or in flight mode when sleeping.

❋ **Choose a bed that's made from natural materials**: if it's wood, make sure it's treated with natural stain, paint and/or wax.

❋ **Invest in a mattress, duvet and pillows that are made from natural materials**: wool is flame- and dustmite-resistant, non-allergenic and antibacterial, without any added chemicals. When buying feather and down, look for cruelty-free options (you may have to ask about this).

❋ **Choose organic cotton or linen sheets**: avoid anything that's labelled as anti-wrinkle; it's more likely to contain chemicals.

❋ **Don't keep any wireless or electrical devices in the bedroom**, including your Wi-Fi router or a TV. If you do have any electrical equipment in there, turn it off when you sleep.

❉ **Keep your bed away from any wall that may have electrical objects on the other side of it.**

❉ **Don't use any chemical oils or synthetic lubricants during sex** that might interfere with hormones or pheromones. Use a natural lube or coconut oil.

❉ **Look after your teeth by brushing them twice a day,** flossing and going for regular dental checks, and by treating any gum or respiratory infection. Infections in the mouth, as well as the sinuses, ears, nose and throat, can affect the reproductive tract if you practise oral sex.

Weeks 10 and 11: going deeper

Every day I am becoming healthier, wiser,
happier and more fertile and cultivating love for myself.

By now you are on track with your practical pillars: you have found the food that works for TCP, you manage 150 minutes of exercise a week (most weeks!), and your home and lifestyle are becoming increasingly natural. This fortnight is about tackling stress in new ways and going a little deeper into your emotions, your trauma and your lived experiences.

Your conception journal

This fortnight you'll be working on the theme of the Mother Wound trauma (see Chapter 5).

Your journaling prompts
Explore your relationship with your mother and the relationship that she had with her own mother, from what you know.

❉ What ideas or prejudices were passed down or inherited from your maternal line? And what hardships or circumstances in that lineage may have led to these ideas or values?

❋ Where in your life do you feel confined or cornered?

❋ Do you feel you've outgrown the labels assigned to you, or certain aspects of your life, and sense an overwhelming need for change? Do you feel resentful in any part of your life where you may have thought you needed to subscribe to a certain way of being, in order to appease your parents?

❋ Do you find it difficult to communicate your needs and desires?

❋ How do you feel about becoming a mother or father?

❋ Do you believe that success only comes from hard work and challenges?

❋ Do you have negative associations with being a woman or a man, and do you notice yourself having any prejudice towards each gender?

❋ How were the women in your lineage treated by men? Is there a history of abuse, either with you or with other women in your lineage?

❋ What is your relationship like with the opposite sex?

❋ Do you find it hard accepting that something could come easily to you, and feel more comfortable being met with challenge or difficulty?

Journaling exercise: healing words

You may already have discovered that writing about trauma can be very healing. The authority on this, the psychologist professor James W. Pennebaker, author of *Expressive Writing: Words that Heal*, has shown that releasing your thoughts and feelings on paper about a stressful, emotional or traumatic experience eases pent-up emotional stress and improves both mental and physical health. His exercise is a specific way of doing this. One of the people Pennebaker trained, who had suffered abuse as a child and poor health as an adult, had a 50 per cent reduction in the number of hospital visits after doing this exercise.

How to do it: set aside fifteen to twenty minutes a day, four days in a row, to write about an issue. When you write, state the issue in question. Then describe what happened. Next describe how it felt then, and how it feels now. Finally depict the impact it's had on your life.

Daily meditation

Heart-chakra activation

This chakra helps us to cultivate compassion and self-love, as well as love for others. When it's activated, it becomes a channel through which infinite love can flow and healing can take place in our most vulnerable areas. Crystals that you can use include rose quartz, emerald, green aventurine, amazonite and malachite.

* Close your eyes and take deep breaths in and out.

* Place both hands over your heart and bring your awareness to the space that surrounds your heart, rising and falling with each breath. Breathe in and out through this area.

* Feel the rhythm of your heart pulsing underneath your hands.

* Visualize an emerald-green light in this area beginning to get warmer, then expanding and rising up your chest.

* See a person you love in front of you and allow yourself to emanate love from your heart to this person.

* Do the same with someone you've had a difficult relationship with (this could be your mother).

* And, finally, see yourself in front of you and emanate love towards yourself.

* Breathe in gratitude and love and send it all around your body as you breathe out and into your aura.

* Breathe in respect and compassion and send it all around your body as you breathe out and into your aura.

* Breathe in the feeling of being a parent and holding your child, and send it all around your body as you breathe out and into your aura.

* Say out loud:

  ○ I am love, and love is all aspects of me.

  ○ I am worthy of receiving infinite love and blessings.

  ○ I am deserving of my dream and of being loved.

  ○ I cultivate gentleness, compassion and gratitude for myself and my circumstances.

  ○ All my relationships are loving and harmonious.

* Bring your attention to your breath and slowly open your eyes, becoming aware of your surroundings.

Loving-kindness meditation

Most of us are our own worst critics. Often that criticism stems from messages we internalized from our parents or from the world as we grew up. This meditation is another technique to combat this kind of baked-in negativity. When you notice criticism of yourself creeping in, stop and pay attention to where it seems to be coming from. Ask yourself, 'Whose voice is this? Would I speak to my best friend with these words, or in that tone?' Each time you stop and reflect, it will become easier to autocorrect yourself. Finally, instead of criticizing yourself, find words of comfort, loving-kindness and compassion for yourself. For example, 'I am doing the best I can in the circumstances, and I'm going to stop being so hard on myself.'

Togetherness: shared emotions

Sometimes, on the face of things, a couple appears to be committed to having a child together, but they both have unspoken and unprocessed emotion that is interfering with this. As we saw in Chapter 5, dealing with trauma can require the help of an experienced counsellor, therapist or sexologist. However, the techniques outlined in that chapter can be beneficial and may help you cultivate a better mind–body connection with yourself. These are some lovely practices to do together:

* **Explore whatever you feel grateful for in your relationship;** then explore where you feel your needs weren't met. See if you can engage in finding solutions together.

* **Practise expressing and vocalizing your needs**, taking turns with your partner. This will help ease your nervous system out of suppression mode.

* **Gradually practise leaning into more of what you're both feeling**: joy as well as discomfort. Recognize the emotions coming up and give yourself full permission to feel them, without judgement. Then notice where in your body you feel the emotion most intensely and see if you can tap into the wisdom of what your body is wishing to tell you, and what it needs. Recognize that any judgement or doubt is probably suppression by the part of your mind that wants you to continue doing what you were doing, in order to keep you safe and protect you. Appreciate that it will feel hard and counterintuitive at first for both of you.

MINDFUL MOVEMENT: YOGA

Yoga can be especially powerful for fertility. It helps you return to the present by regulating your breath while you practise challenging poses. It opens up a space to witness and observe any negative patterns of your thoughts on autopilot. The physical exertion of holding and moving through some of the poses can trigger a sense of over-whelm, but as you learn to bear this, you rewire your brain to become more resilient and develop your ability to bear difficult emotions too.

Retrain your stress system

It sounds counterintuitive, but small intermittent bursts of stress can work to counter the effects of chronic stress. This is the effect known as hormesis. However, only use such short stressors if and when you feel you have the emotional and mental capacity to handle them. Ideally they should be done when you feel relaxed, otherwise they simply act as additional stressors. Avoid doing them in the second half or luteal phase of the cycle, when you're most sensitive to cortisol. And make sure it's safe for you to do the physical elements by checking with your doctor if you have an existing medical condition.

Some suggestions for benefiting from hormesis are:

* **Have cold showers and consider cold-water swimming:** this can increase levels of immune cells and the production of mitochondria, increase longevity and lower inflammation. Recent research shows that women who do this before pregnancy may have improved obstetric outcomes.

* **Do high-intensity interval training:** this involves intermittent bursts of all the exercise you can do for thirty seconds, followed by a rest period of fifteen seconds, stimulating the production of mitochondria (see Chapter 7 for advice on this, because it isn't for everyone and should be modified in pregnancy).

* **Engage in mental challenges,** such as preparing a presentation or learning a new hobby. This can activate

beneficial cellular mechanisms, including the production of a brain chemical that promotes neuroplasticity in the central nervous system.

CRYSTALS FOR FERTILITY

Crystals are energy medicine in solid form. You can meditate with them next to you, by placing them on the chakras they feel most aligned to, as in the chakra activations. You can sleep with them under your pillow or next to your bed. Or you can wear them as jewellery, or even put them in your bra.

Shiva lingam: This stone is sourced from the holy Narmada River in India, which represents the divine masculine and feminine. It activates sexual energies and helps to realign all the energetic centres.

Carnelian: this aligns with the sacral chakra, helping to ground you and stimulating a feeling of sensuality, strength and joy. Its warm colour links it to courage.

Clear quartz: this crystal amplifies the energetic field and the effectiveness of our thoughts, so it's useful to keep it nearby. It also has a positive effect on the endocrine and nervous systems.

Rose quartz: traditionally used for fertility, this works with the heart centre, opening us up to love and compassion and overcoming painful feelings and issues.

Moonstone: this reflects the qualities of the moon, helping to stabilize emotions. It is also linked with female health and fertility, so it can help with a range of female disorders. It is often seen as a stone for lovers, helping to enhance intuition and spiritual guidance.

Cycle monitoring: understanding your personal fertility

Now that you're nearly three months into cycle monitoring, you'll have begun to see how your energy and mood change over the course of the month. Below is a guide to how fluctuating hormones affect most women, and how to adapt to these patterns so that you can live in greater alignment with them.

Follicular phase

This is when you feel most energetic and creative. Focus on starting new projects, solving problems and dealing with challenging situations or conflict. You'll be open to new experiences at this time and to socializing too.

During ovulation

You're at your most communicative and outward-focused, so this is the time to take on big conversations, presentations and first dates. As you are at your most fertile now, you may find you're more drawn towards feeling and looking your best.

Luteal phase

Your body is calling for nurturing, attention and comfort, so you may find that you're more focused on domestic life rather than your social life. This is also a time when you may feel more perceptive, especially in the few days before your period. Any difficult feelings that surface at this time are a good indication of what may have been bothering you, but which you may have concealed and suppressed. This is a great time to rest and replenish with self-care rituals.

During menstruation

You're called to go inwards now. This is a great time to reflect and self-evaluate, to allow yourself to experience your emotions and listen to your instincts. Writing down these feelings and thought patterns will provide insight into issues that need changing or situations that require processing. Your body communicates most powerfully to you at this time, and you'll find it's a good time for self-care. If your emotions are feeling triggered, call on those you trust to support you. This will help you to cultivate a trusting relationship with yourself too.

Week 12: reflection

My body is getting ready to welcome new life.

You have done so well: twelve whole weeks of focusing on yourself (and on your relationship with your partner, if you have one). This week you'll continue with your affirmations and activations while reflecting on what you've achieved, as well as how you want to continue to practise TCP.

Your conception journal

Your journaling prompts

* Reflect back on the relationship you had with your own parents.

* What do you feel, or wish, could have been different in what they did? Or in their relationship with you?

* What do you wish they could have been like?

* Does that change how you feel about becoming a parent? How?

* Does that make you think of anything you can keep working on to become the parent you hope your child will have?

* What kind of parent would you like to be?

* Is there more that you'd like to change before a child enters your life?

* What can you do now to become the parent that you hope your child will have?

Daily meditation

Throat-chakra activation

The throat chakra is the most important communication centre of the body. It's responsible for self-expression as well as for communicating your truth, needs and desires. As it lies between the heart and the head, it's also a mediator between thoughts and emotions. Activation of this area will help in being able to express yourself as fully, expansively and compassionately as possible. Crystals that you can use include kyanite, lapis lazuli, aquamarine, blue-lace agate and blue apatite.

* On your hands and knees, arch your back and go into a cat pose, then hollow your back into a cow pose.

* Open your mouth and stick out your tongue, stretching it towards your chin.

* As you exhale, draw the sound 'Ha' from your abdomen and repeat this a few times.

* Come out of the pose and sit.

* Close your eyes and take some deep breaths in and out.

* Visualize the colour blue in your throat, getting brighter and expanding, filling your throat with purity and cleansing.

* As you exhale, let go of any stress or tension you've been holding there.

* Let the colour blue spread out from your body and into your aura.

* As you breathe out, chant the word 'Ham' and let the sound carry on for the entire duration of the exhale.

* As you feel the vibration, sense that any obstacles are being released from your throat.

* Gently tapping on the area between your collar bones, say these affirmations out loud:

- o I feel free to speak my truth and express how I feel.

- o I use my words consciously to bring positive change in the world.

- o I release all fears and limitations that stop me from expressing my truth.

- o I set clear boundaries that align with who I am.

- o I am balanced and compassionate when communicating with others.

- o I speak with authenticity and grace.

Bring your awareness to your breath, open your eyes and draw your attention back to your surroundings.

SPEAKING OUT

This week's activation is about the throat chakra and speaking out. Expressing yourself has a primal link to the pelvic area, and therefore to fertility too. Physiotherapists recognize that there's a strong jaw–pelvis connection. Improving the mobility of the jaw can unleash tension in the pelvis, and vice versa. I have noticed that women who suffer with problems in their pelvis can often have a problem expressing their emotions and verbalizing what they're feeling, and this can often relate back to trauma experiences earlier in their lives.

If we go back to how the human foetus develops, we can see this isn't coincidence. At around day 15 of foetal development, the membrane that forms the mouth (oropharyngeal) develops at the same time as the membrane that forms the urinary, digestive and reproductive tracts (cloacal). The spine forms between them – and they remain connected.

A final reflection exercise to end the 12-week plan

Look back at the beginning of your journal to reflect on how far you've come. Who was the person you were when you started this plan? How are you different now? What has changed externally in your life? And what has changed internally, in terms of how you feel and behave? You may be surprised by how big the changes are, in lots of different aspects. I often describe this effect as a client having given birth to themselves.

Often people begin to look, act and even sound different after TCP – to the point where others will notice the differences and wonder what they're doing! People also often become more energetic, have improved concentration and feel healthier. What I've also noticed, which is no coincidence, is that they become incredibly powerful manifesters, upgrading so many different elements of their life.

Some changes make other people feel uncomfortable, but don't worry if this is the case for you. When you follow a path of healing you are going to leave some people behind as you grow into a different person – the parent you wish to become. You will make new friends and deepen some bonds too, because far more people will be inspired by this. Those who are not ready to see you change are probably those who are no longer aligned with you, because you've grown to become the truest and most authentic version of yourself.

You might be behaving differently in relationships, and even being a different sort of person at work too. People describe making different decisions, being better at setting boundaries, recognizing the need to take time out for themselves and to prioritize self-care by listening to the messages their body is sending out. They even step away from jobs they no longer feel aligned to, or may decide to go after a dream they want to achieve. One client transformed the way she dressed, switching from neutral colours to brights she naturally felt drawn to.

Now reflect on everything you've achieved in this three-month period.

Conclusion to the 12-week plan

This has been twelve weeks very well spent. You have overhauled your lifestyle in the areas you need to improve, investing in your long-term health and wellness.

If you've been following TCP with the thought of trying to conceive in the future, please keep using what you've learned. If you have a gynaecological condition, you may have noticed that TCP has alleviated your symptoms (see Part 3 of the book).

If you've been trying to get pregnant, doing TCP has made it more likely that you will become so (or you may already be pregnant) and has helped improve the health of your future child. You have made a significant investment in your own long-term health and well-being, and have brought a new consciousness to the idea of being a parent.

I hope you feel more confident about where you are in your fertility journey, even if you haven't yet conceived. Your eggs (or sperm) will have improved their condition, and the whole environment in your body will be more conducive to conception. I hope this gives you optimism for the future: you have the power to control much of your health and can tap into the power of your epigenome with these targeted, slow and sustainable changes.

Your body and mind have changed in a positive way, and you are probably fitter and healthier and more emotionally attuned. You have become closer to the kind of parent and person you want to be, and that is what matters.

How to continue TCP

* **Continue your new eating and exercise habits:** they are healthy for the long term.

* **Keep on replacing products and foods with natural alternatives,** and be aware of how you can keep your toxin exposure to a minimum.

THE CONCEPTION PLAN

		Week 1	Weeks 2 & 3	Weeks 4 & 5
	THE FIVE PILLARS	Continue actioning the changes suggested across the five pillars: Nutrition, Exercise, Stress management, Toxin-free living, Sex and relationships. Use your journal to plan these into your weeks.		
THE 12-WEEK PLAN	**YOUR CONCEPTION JOURNAL**	Journal exercises: try to write in your journal every day of the 12-week plan. This can be free writing, a gratitude diary, a letter, affirmations, a dream diary or inspired by the journal prompts suggested each week.		
	DAILY MEDITATION	Third-eye chakra activation (page 150)	Solar-plexus chakra activation (page 156) Mindful-thought detox (page 157)	Crown-chakra activation (page 163)
	DAILY VISUALIZATION	Spend five minutes each day visualizing yourself as a parent already (page 151).		
	FOCUS AREAS	The basics (page 151) Self-care (page 152)	Toxin-free living (page 159)	Breathwork: Deepening the connection with yourself (page 165)
	CYCLE MONITORING	Start tracking your cycle (page 153)	Notice any abnormalities in your cycle (page 158)	Exercise in tune with your cycle (page 164)
PERSONALIZATION		Use Part 3 of the book to customize your plan, depending on any conditions or considerations you may have.		

Weeks 6 & 7	Weeks 8 & 9	Weeks 10 & 11	Week 12
Continue actioning the changes suggested across the five pillars: Nutrition, Exercise, Stress management, Toxin-free living, Sex and relationships. Use your journal to plan these into your weeks.			
Feelings check-in: each day of the 12-week plan do a feelings check-in, writing your responses in your journal and seeing how they change (page 149).			
Sacral-chakra activation (page 168)	Root-chakra activation (page 176)	Heart-chakra activation (page 187) Loving-kindness meditation (page 188)	Throat-chakra activation (page 194)
Spend five minutes each day visualizing yourself as a parent already (page 151).			
Focus on food (page 168) Revive with self-care (page 174)	Focus on pleasure (page 178) Focus on relationships (page 181) Bedroom detox (page 184)	Togetherness (page 189) Retrain your stress system (page 190)	Final reflection exercise (page 196)
Eat in tune with your cycle (page 171)	Sex to suit your cycle (page 177)	Understanding your personal fertility (page 192)	
Use Part 3 of the book to customize your plan, depending on any conditions or considerations you may have.			

✳ **Make sure you allow time for yourself each day**, and time for your relationship too.

✳ **Pick the activations, journaling prompts and affirmations** that you feel most drawn to. If you identified any specific areas that need addressing or particular energetic centres, when working on yourself or with a therapist, focusing on those would be a good idea. If you only have time for one thing each day, write down a daily moment of gratitude (see page 148).

✳ **If you have been diagnosed with any health conditions**, or you have experienced a miscarriage, or you are older or are starting ART, or you want to encourage your partner to do TCP (if he hasn't already), Part 3 of the book explains how to customize TCP with additional, specialized elements, going forward.

Ideally you want to be continuing TCP, and adapting it, right into your pregnancy and beyond. It's a set of principles and values that you should adopt for the rest of your life. Doing this work will help you deepen your own intuition and understanding about whether you want to continue trying to get pregnant naturally or seek additional help. Consulting a doctor and getting their guidance is an important part of this, but the decision always lies with you and has to feel aligned with your own values and your authentic truth, which the preceding work will have helped you to become clearer on.

PART 3
Personalizing TCP to you

Introduction

Part 3 is for you if you've picked up this book because you have a gynae-cological condition that you're worried may be affecting your ability to get pregnant – or may threaten to do so in the future. Or you may have another life factor that is looming large in your worries about getting pregnant, such as your age, or you may have been told you might need IVF. This part of the book gives you some more specialized advice on how to make TCP work for specific challenges and circumstances.

But first there's a chapter for male partners. Of course the whole of TCP is for men, but this chapter discusses sperm health and other issues that affect men in depth. Then, very importantly, there's a chapter on baby loss (including an unsuccessful IVF cycle or an early miscarriage) and where TCP may be of help. Chapter 13 is for you if you're over the age of thirty-five, because it can feel like a significant milestone if you're not pregnant by this point (and even more so if you are over the age of forty). Chapter 14 is TCP advice if you're considering or are already having assisted conception, because the world of IVF clinics can be a hard one to negotiate through a holistic lens. In each of these chapters I include the advice that I give to clients, for you to consider in addition to any advice you may get from your own doctor. And there are spiritually and emotionally healing ways to approach each issue, and suggestions for ways to personalize the TCP advice.

The final five chapters of the book are about reproductive condi-tions that affect fertility. You'll see that I have a different approach from most doctors – one that integrates all the aspects of what might con-tribute to a condition, including the emotional and energetic aspects. I developed TCP as the result of seeing many patients alleviate their symptoms and conceive from this starting point. This section covers how trauma and suppressed emotions, which you learned about in Part 1, affect the female body. It explains how they can manifest as many different conditions that can impact on fertility, including the most common ones, such as PCOS and endometriosis. In these chapters you will explore how to adapt TCP to your condition, as well as how to consider your condition from a new perspective: as something you can manage and influence, rather than being reliant on external sources.

CHAPTER 11

TCP for male infertility

It's difficult and often a shock to be told that your sperm may not get your partner pregnant. 'It's a real blow to your sense of self,' Jay says. 'There's a niggling voice in the back of your head telling you you've failed your manliness test; please hand in your testicles at reception.' In a 2017 survey, 93 per cent of men said that infertility had a negative impact on their well-being and self-esteem, making them feel depressed, anxious, lonely and even suicidal.

At the same time as this emotional challenge, you may feel the burden of supporting your partner and/or guilt that she is the one who's having more invasive investigations and is facing the brunt of any fertility treatment. You may feel isolated in your grief, confusion and anger, coupled with perceiving yourself as falling short of the culturally endorsed virile version of manhood. You may also have been conditioned not to want to appear incapable or weak, compounding the pressure that you're putting on yourself.

You are not the only man in this position. In fact, far from it: you're one of millions around the world who are struggling with infertility. Modern life has led to men not only having lower testosterone levels, but also a critical reduction in sperm numbers as well as quality. Male infertility now makes up 40–50 per cent of overall infertility. Fertility in men is decreasing each year by 1 per cent – dubbed the '1 per cent effect' – along with miscarriage rates increasing in women (miscarriage is, in part, contributed to by poor sperm quality).

Some of this may have happened early in life – in fact in the womb. Male foetuses are particularly vulnerable to the effects of environmental toxins. In the womb, a baby's reproductive system is epigenetically programmed, which will have a continuing effect on the fertility of future generations. Key times are conception and during the first trimester, when the testicles and the cells that will become sperm later in life are being formed, as well as straight after birth (the other key window in a man's life is adolescence).

Research shows that if a mother smokes while pregnant, this reduces sperm counts in male children by 40 per cent, and a mother's stress has been shown to have an impact too. Over the last couple of decades there has been a rise in a constellation of abnormalities referred to as testicular dysgenesis syndrome: genitourinary abnormalities, infertility and testicular cancer. There has also been a rise in Klinefelter syndrome, a chromosomal condition with an absence of sperm, which is now thought to be due in part to epigenetic abnormalities in both the mother and the father. The fact that these conditions are increasing suggests there is something environmental, and not simply genetic, behind rising rates of male infertility.

There is another important reason, outside of conception, why male infertility matters: your health. It's been associated with a higher chance of chronic conditions such as diabetes, ischaemic heart disease, testicular and prostate cancer, along with a greater risk of dying earlier in life. Having healthy sperm parameters appears to be a barometer of overall health and to provide important insights into your long-term well-being.

Why sperm quality matters

There is one misconception I want to tackle immediately: good sperm does not equal manliness. I have seen young, fit men attend for a semen analysis, only to find their sperm parameters are abnormally low. As many as one in two men has sperm that don't meet the normal range, at least in some measurements.

Prostatic fluid (a fluid that sperm is exposed to) and sperm depend on a number of different hormones secreted by various endocrine glands across the body. These include growth hormone from the pituitary gland, DHEA (dehydroepiandrosterone) from the adrenals, melatonin from the pineal gland and TRH (thyrotrophin-releasing hormone) from the thyroid. An imbalance in any one of these can have direct effects on male fertility, as can factors that also affect the brain and adrenals, such as mental and physical stress.

Sperm quality is measured by concentration (how many), morphology (normality), motility (how fast) and vitality (whether they're alive). If a man has one of these in a range below normal, he has twice the risk of infertility compared to someone who meets the normal criteria. If all of them are below normal, this goes up exponentially to sixteen times the risk.

Men produce around 300 million new sperm a day, and each ejaculation contains around 100 million sperm, so you'd assume that any drop in quality wouldn't matter. Yet it does. The egg uses a trail of chemical signals in its surrounding follicular fluid to attract the most genetically compatible sperm, and it's estimated that only 250 make it to the egg. By then, quality really does matter. And if a sperm with a high degree of DNA damage does fertilize the egg, the chances of an embryo surviving and developing normally are low.

A semen analysis doesn't tell you everything about sperm function or wholly predict male reproductive capacity. The 'normal' values in a semen analysis don't reflect average values, but are based on a minimum standard for pregnancy. And so 15 per cent of men with 'normal' sperm results may also have suboptimal fertility.

There is another test to look at sperm quality called 'DNA fragmentation testing', because men with infertility have a greater extent of DNA damage and lower sperm-DNA integrity. Many clinics don't necessarily offer this test, but instead use ICSI (intracytoplasmic sperm injection, a method whereby sperm is injected into an egg cell to achieve fertilization – more detail on this later) to help overcome any issues relating to fertilization.

However, ICSI may not always be the best solution. The rate of miscarriage, along with chromosomal abnormalities in the baby, is higher after conception via ICSI. Having ICSI means that, potentially, compromised sperm may end up leading to conception and may confer various adverse factors on the future child, leading to chronic health issues later in life, as well as possible future problems with their own fertility. Testing for DNA fragmentation may give you greater insight into your infertility, as well as the chance to track any improvements through lifestyle or other interventions.

Even if you end up having ICSI, it's still important to improve the overall condition of sperm DNA, so that it's optimized prior to conception. One study reported that IVF or ICSI with high levels of DNA damage had more than twice the risk of early pregnancy loss.

It takes just under three months for sperm to mature fully. Sperm DNA is prone to mutations caused by its environment, which is probably an evolutionary survival mechanism. This means that sperm are prone to positive influences too. Because sperm turnover is so frequent, TCP can help create a new environment and can reprogramme sperm and reproductive capacities within twelve weeks, although it may take longer in some cases (and some men may need medical or surgical help too).

TCP for male fertility

Sperm environment

Factors besides recognized chemical toxins will affect your fertility. These include wireless electromagnetic radiation and heat (tight underwear or trousers, long-distance driving, hot tubs or electric blankets). Sperm can also be affected by oxidative stress caused by a poor diet, alcohol, smoking, supplementation of testosterone and other steroids, some medications, chronic prostate infections and varicoceles (see below). The combination of many of these hormone-disrupting stressors is thought to lie behind rising instances of testicular dysgenesis syndrome, as well as contributing to adverse epigenetic effects on the rest of the male reproductive tract.

Age

After the age of forty, testosterone levels gradually reduce – this is known as the andropause. Testosterone is key not only to libido and preventing erectile dysfunction, but also to sperm quality. Rather than taking testosterone supplements, which can reduce fertility, there are other ways to support the production of your own testosterone naturally. Looking after your overall health (as in TCP) will do this, as well as affecting epigenetic mechanisms that may help delay the onset of the andropause and mitigate the impact of low testosterone.

Although a man can still biologically father a child into older age, sperm are likely to have more DNA damage and more chromosomal abnormalities, leading to lower rates of fertilization and an increased risk of congenital abnormalities in the baby, as well as higher rates of autism and schizophrenia and of miscarriage. In couples who have recurrent miscarriages, men appear to have sperm with twice the normal level of DNA fragmentation. It has been shown that, generally speaking, older fathers pass on far more random genetic mutations compared to older mothers.

However, older fathers also happen to pass on longer telomeres, the caps on DNA that protect the genetic information, and this may give rise to children who live longer. And because a lot of DNA damage to sperm comes from oxidative stress, lifestyle measures such as those in TCP that help to counter this can not only increase sperm quality, but also imprint a child with healthier, longer life prospects and may even enhance their intelligence.

Erectile dysfunction (ED)

CASE STUDY

Like many other men, Tony found it difficult to discuss his ED. Not only was it affecting the relationship with his wife and making it difficult to conceive, but it was also affecting his confidence. Tony was someone who tended to internalize his feelings, for fear of judgement, which would sometimes find an outlet in bursts of anger. As he was talking about his story, he noticed that his right foot began to twitch and he realized this was the same foot he'd used in a moment of frustration, to smash a glass door with. It was potentially a sign of the repressed memories of trauma that he was storing there.

Once Tony realized the power of identifying and dealing with his emotions, he became curious about what the ED was wanting to show him about all the unexpressed parts of himself, and he came to see it as an ally, rather than meeting it with resistance. He claimed that 'it opened the doors of my personality', so that he was finally free to explore the fullness of himself, without judgement. He started practising mindfulness and meditation to bring acceptance to all the parts that had previously been buried and suppressed and that were creating internal stress. He began to share this with his wife, who supported and encouraged him through it, which deepened the connection between them.

Ultimately Tony realized that his ED helped to forge a new relationship with himself, whereby he started to become increasingly comfortable with his feelings, understanding that his body was a vehicle and a means of calling him to action over his own previously neglected emotional needs. And as he brought emotional healing to himself, he started to notice how this translated into physical benefits too.

ED affects older men more than younger men, although nearly one-third of ED affects men under the age of forty-five. If it happens from time to time, it isn't necessarily a cause for concern. But if it happens regularly, it will start to affect your sexual relationship and your self-esteem, as well as the chances of conception, and will provide useful clues into some wider health issues. Aside from low testosterone levels, other factors contribute to ED, including diabetes and poor blood flow, alcohol and/or smoking. And, as Tony's case study demonstrates, emotional factors too.

If you experience ED regularly, you need to be investigated for physiological causes. Medical treatment is usually oral medication (phosphodiesterase type-5 inhibitors or Viagra), but also penile pumps, implants, penile injections and intraurethral (in the urethra) medication. Lifestyle factors, such as exercise, are key too: losing weight if you're obese, eating healthily, addressing stress and relationship issues, as well as abstaining from alcohol and smoking.

ED can also be associated with premature ejaculation. The fear of losing an erection may cause you to want to hurry, and the stress contributing to ED may impact on ejaculation too. Consuming porn regularly interferes with arousal circuits and can lead to ED as well as to premature ejaculation. For the latter, pelvic-floor exercises may help, and sometimes medication too. But as with many reproductive issues, emotional patterns often contribute.

Emotions

Just as female fertility problems can be rooted in stress, suppressed emotions and trauma, so those of men can be too. On top of this, men often have fewer opportunities to discuss emotional (and fertility) issues.

In clinic, I often see a disconnect between how a man feels on the inside and the masculine identity that he projects on the outside, due to societal, family and even his partner's expectations. Feeling unable to express your feelings or having to conform to society's distorted version of what a man is may have left you feeling powerless and disconnected from your truth from a young age. This can be compounded by failing to conceive. Resentment and anger can build up in the body, specifically in the reproductive tissues.

I often see men who feel a real pressure, and need, to be in control and who aren't comfortable being intimate because they feel unable to confront their emotions. Or who are self-critical and self-blaming. There are also links to Mother Wound trauma (see Chapter 5) if, as a child, you felt powerless or couldn't protect your mother, or you were told not to cry or show your feelings. Or you may have had to step into the role of being a man early in life in order to provide or protect, or had an overbearing mother, or were a victim of sexual, physical or verbal bullying or abuse. Some men also experience unresolved conflict over having children if they fear that what happened to them will happen again, or self-doubt over being able to manage fatherhood, which they can find difficult to acknowledge.

Other issues

Other issues that can affect sperm production include: childhood infections such as mumps; undescended testicles; chronic and chromosomal disease; and various toxins. Low numbers or no sperm in the ejaculate can be due to an obstruction in the tubes that the sperm travel through. Varicoceles are very common in men who have abnormal sperm parameters, affecting 40 per cent of those with infertility. These are swollen veins or varices in the testicles and may impact on sperm production by interfering with blood flow and increasing the temperature of the scrotum.

Research into the testicular microbiome is helping us to understand another cause behind male infertility; it seems that a lack of microbial diversity, and more pathogenic bacteria as a result of unhealthier habits, are linked to low sperm counts or having no sperm. Not only may this knowledge lead to new testing and therapies, but it may also help to better predict which men will benefit from surgical sperm retrieval, a technique that is used when a man has an obstruction that stops sperm getting out in the usual way. Sperm is then either frozen or used in fertility treatment such as ICSI (for more on this, see page 254).

How to adapt TCP for male fertility

If you commit to the 12-week plan, TCP may help boost natural testosterone, improve DNA integrity and optimize sperm parameters. You can also customize TCP with the following suggestions:

* **Expose your scrotum to sunlight** to increase the production of vitamin D, which in turn will stimulate the production of sperm.

* **Take probiotics and eat probiotic foods** to help support natural levels of minerals such as zinc and selenium, which support good sperm production. Probiotics also optimize the seminal microbiome, which is emerging as an important component of male reproductive health.

* **Reduce the amount of soya in your diet** to keep oestrogen levels low.

* **Consider a good supplement with a range of antioxidants**, such as vitamins B, C, D and E, as well as zinc, selenium, coenzyme Q10 and N-acetyl cysteine.

* **Consider taking the herbs ashwagandha and maca root under the direction of a herbalist**; both have been shown to improve libido.

❈ **Reduce the amount of refined sugar in your diet** as it can lead to increased conversion of testosterone to oestrogen, which impacts negatively on infertility.

❈ **Use methods to reduce inflammation and oxidative stress,** whether through diet, exercise or stress management, to help promote the production of growth hormone. This is significant for sperm development, as well as overseeing sugar control, the thyroid and parathyroid hormones and the adrenal hormones. So it's important to support the natural production of growth hormone, especially in older men, in whom it tends to decline after the age of thirty.

❈ **Keep electromagnetic radiation around your testicles low;** don't carry your mobile phone in your pocket for long periods.

❈ **Avoid extreme heat;** sperm production requires cooler temperatures, so avoid wearing tight or restrictive underwear, saunas, hot tubs or regular baths, driving for prolonged periods of time and hot environments.

❈ **I strongly recommend that you stop smoking** (even e-cigarettes, although the evidence for this is not yet established) because it can cause damage to sperm that may even be passed on to the baby. Second-hand smoke inhalation by a pregnant woman can negatively affect the growth and development of the child.

❈ **A medical condition such as hypertension or heart disease may affect your fertility** and it's important to get this under control before embarking on conception. Check with your doctor about any long-term medication you may be on that could affect your sperm count or quality.

❈ **If you need to use lubrication during intercourse,** aim for natural oils, such as coconut or mineral oil, rather than synthetic ones, which can contain harmful chemicals.

✳ **Do regular exercise** to help spike growth-hormone levels naturally, especially cardiovascular exercise and weights.

✳ **Try whole-body massage with your partner** and direct sensual stimulation of the penis, to help boost sex drive as well as natural testosterone levels.

✳ **Abstain from porn,** as this has been shown to lead to desensitization in both men and women and problems with sexual dynamics.

✳ **Have sex often and throughout your partner's menstrual cycle**; recent studies suggest that sperm quality may actually improve with more regular sex, increasing the chance of conception, and can also help to protect against prostate cancer.

✳ **Don't neglect your emotional needs**; whether its dealing with your own infertility or helping to support your partner, seek assistance from a counsellor or a support group if you need it, for helpful strategies as well as for knowing that you are not alone. Mind—body therapies can be extremely beneficial, especially for men who aren't necessarily comfortable articulating their emotions.

Journaling prompts

✳ Do you feel anxious a lot of the time, and what are your anxieties about?

✳ Do you place unfair burdens on yourself, and how does this make you feel?

✳ What resentments do you hold and where do they stem from?

✳ Do you struggle to express your own needs, and do you tend to compensate by being too controlling?

❋ Where does the need to appear strong and dominant come from, and how has it affected your relationships?

❋ What was your relationship with your mother and father like?

❋ What circumstances did you face in life that might have been traumatic and have left you feeling less of a man?

❋ Does being vulnerable scare you and, if so, why?

❋ Where are you self-sabotaging, and what's leading you to do this?

❋ Where have you taken on too many responsibilities in life? Where do you have anxieties about living up to expectations, and what contributed to this?

❋ How does it make you feel when other people are reliant on you?

❋ Are you living in alignment with your core values and beliefs and, if not, why not?

❋ Who may have tried to control or challenge your authority, and how did it leave you feeling?

❋ What are your true feelings about fatherhood?

CHAPTER 12

TCP for miscarriage and baby loss

From the moment you think you've conceived it's impossible not to let your mind project into the future. The feeling of becoming a mother – of bringing new life into the world – is a combination of hope, happiness and excitement.

The emotional bond that women feel with their children, even before they're born, is more than just psychological. This process of becoming a mother has a name: matrescence. There are real biological transformations happening; hormonal and neurological changes prepare the brain for the behavioural, emotional and mental tasks of being a caregiver. The brain starts to remodel with new central-nervous-system circuits, expanding a woman's emotional capacity and sensitivity (and bringing heightened emotions too). Research shows that these brain changes may even have a protective effect on brain function later in life.

Sadly, for many women this process stops unexpectedly short. Baby loss affects one in four people and potentially more, as many early losses are not necessarily recognized. If you have been one of them, you'll probably have been told some of the facts already: miscarriage is more common than flu, and most miscarriages take place in the first trimester.

But this chapter isn't only about what is usually recognized as a miscarriage. When I talk about 'baby loss', I include silent miscarriage, where the only sign is a heavier period than normal; and a biochemical pregnancy that shows up as a faintly positive pregnancy test, only to disappear soon afterwards. I also include pregnancies that are ectopic (outside the womb cavity), molar (abnormal fertilization) and anembryonic (a pregnancy sac in the womb without an embryo); IVF cycles that fail; and terminations of pregnancy that may take place for a variety of reasons. In fact although society may not recognize or validate your loss, the process of trying for pregnancy that ends with a menstrual bleed instead is a loss that deserves to be honoured as such. That's not to minimize the visceral trauma of losing a longer-term pregnancy, but it is to acknowledge that each person will have their own pain and grief from whatever form of baby loss they may have experienced. And their pain needs, and deserves, to be validated.

The end of any kind of pregnancy, however brief, feels at once unfair, unjust, harrowing and tragic. The loss can be physical: bleeding, the disappearance of any physical symptoms such as breast tenderness, and hormonal changes. Seeing blood or tissue and dealing with contractions, if you have them, is difficult and painful. It can be a shock, especially if it occurs out of the blue, and if you don't have anyone with you to help. Aside from the physical symptoms, it's also the loss of a dream, such as what the baby might look like, what kind of mother or father you'll be, plus choosing baby names and all the excitement that comes with the anticipation of a new life.

Facing the grief of baby loss

It's natural to grieve, to feel bereft or numb, to experience rage or despair, to feel desperate or dark or overwhelmed – or, in fact, any combination of these emotions. It takes time and space to process loss.

What can make this harder is that baby loss isn't always acknowledged. It's only recently that people have begun to talk about it. There is little support: for example, there is no law in the UK for miscarriage leave, unlike in New Zealand. I've met many women and their partners who don't feel able to speak freely about it. This can leave you not only grieving, but also questioning if your grief is valid. Please know that it is: the loss of a child is one of the most devastating events you will ever face.

It's also natural to want to find a reason for your miscarriage. Very often women blame themselves, go over and over what they could have done differently. I've had patients who feel guilty for telling people 'too early' that they were pregnant, for having been too hopeful. I even had a patient who blamed herself for drinking too many green juices. Please recognize that you're not to blame. As you'll see below, miscarriages can happen as a result of many complex factors, but they are not your fault.

MICROCHIMERISM AND THE ENERGETIC BODY

The first step of TCP approach to baby loss is to recognize the lasting impact of a pregnancy, however brief. As we saw in Chapter 2, cells that belong to the foetus mix with the mother's, in a process called microchimerism. Within weeks of conception, cells from the mother and baby traffic back and forth across the placenta, meaning that one becomes part of the other. This may explain the unique maternal bond of humans and other animals that grow their babies in the womb. Women who have experienced baby loss often find it comforting when I explain this, and especially that each pregnancy will always be a physical part of them.

The word 'microchimera' derives from a mythical Greek creature with three parts: the head of a lion, the body of a goat and the tail of a serpent. It highlights how a woman can have three cell populations in her body: her mother's, her own and her child's. Research has detected these migrated cells in the mother years later, and that they act to regenerate and heal the mother's body. They may even extend her lifespan; scientists found that 85 per cent of women with detectable cells live to the age of eighty, but only 67 per cent of those without such cells make it to this age.

With each conception, this reservoir of foetal cells in the mother grows, and so cells can transfer between siblings too. All the children that a mother carries will have imprints of each other, whether or not they survive the entire pregnancy. Microchimeric cells may even boost the mother's tolerance of successive pregnancies, meaning that first children may support the success of their future siblings, even if they themselves don't necessarily survive.

You may also find it astonishing to know that the baby's energetic body develops before its physical body. Harold Burr, Professor of Anatomy at Yale University in the 1930s–1950s, proposed that as an embryo grows and organs are developed, it appears to follow an electromagnetic template that helps to direct the body into different systems. Looking at unfertilized salamander eggs, he found that each one contained an electrical axis; he showed that this axis later aligns with the spinal cord of the baby salamander and forms the central nervous system. This provides scientific evidence for what is a commonly held spiritual belief: living beings have an energetic body, and we can continue integrating the information from it all our lives and can access it through the energetic system of chakras and meridians (see page 40).

The second step of TCP approach is to acknowledge that your pain is valid, to speak about it and process it. Whatever your feelings, don't judge yourself. You will not be alone in having them. You may feel any or all of the following: confusion, sadness, anger, jealousy, guilt, shame, emptiness, loneliness and/or a loss of control. And as emotional pain can activate the same cascade of biological reactions as physical pain, you may also suffer from insomnia, headaches or exhaustion. In other words, grief and loss can physically hurt.

I've met people who've tried to silence their emotional pain and carry on, which our society seems to see as a sign of capability and strength. Many people deal with the overwhelm of emotions by distracting themselves with work. Although that may help you cope in the short term, your feelings will not go away. If they aren't processed, they can become harmful. One in three women who lose their baby will go on to develop PTSD in the long term. Four months later, 30–50 per cent have moderate to severe anxiety and 10–15 per cent have moderate to severe depression. After a year those figures are still at 20 per cent for anxiety and 6 per cent for depression. You don't need to share what's happened with everyone, but it's important to share with someone. Each time you speak or confide in someone you trust, you open a door that enables other women to speak about their grief too. You can start off this process with journaling, which allows you to safely express the depth of what you're feeling without any fear of judgement.

The risk of mental-health issues goes up with recurrent miscarriage, which is now classed as two or more miscarriages (it used to be three). Repeated losses can put an incredible strain on women and their partners, causing anxiety, depression, fatigue, irritability, fear, sleep disturbances and lack of concentration. For some women, even having sex in order to conceive can be triggering, because it carries with it the possibility of having to face grief again.

Being pregnant can be an anxious time in itself, but if you become pregnant after loss, the smallest amount of pain or bleeding can be anxiety-provoking. It's normal to become compulsive about monitoring your symptoms as a result of the worry. I've even had patients with no symptoms terrified they might be having a silent miscarriage. People find having frequent ultrasound scans reassuring at first, but this tends to be short-lived. Pregnancy is often spent cycling between hope and despair, so take one day at a time.

What might help with grief after baby loss

* **Lean into the feelings,** when you can, sit with them and allow them to guide you towards what you may need to process. Taking your mind off your grief for a short time may be helpful, but you do need to go through grief in order to heal.

* **Don't judge yourself for what you're feeling** and how long it's taking. Grief is a process without a time limit, and it can be a messy one where you flit between denial, anger, needing to understand and feeling hopelessness. Eventually you will be able to tolerate being reminded of the loss, yet remain present and hopeful.

* **Share with someone you trust or a support group** when you're ready. It's natural to want to take time for yourself

and your partner at first, but sharing may help you feel less alone and may also help another person heal.

* **Remember most people mean well**, even when they say unhelpful things that can be hurtful. As there's little openness or education about baby loss in our society, people struggle to find supportive words. We're all responsible for improving our education around this, but it may be helpful for you to explain how their concern could have been expressed better and where they could have been more supportive, once you have the emotional bandwidth to do so.

* **Be honest about what you need from others**, whether that's time out or avoiding discussions on a subject. If you can, let your boss know, so they can ensure you're not met with a difficult situation on returning to work. And tell your midwife, who can ensure that you're not sent any more reminders of antenatal appointments.

* **Ask your loved ones for practical help with food, shopping or childcare.** Normal tasks such as eating, sleeping and exercising may seem impossible at first, but nurturing yourself is part of healing. Take small steps towards supporting your physical healing; this will become easier over time.

* **Depression, anxiety and PTSD are common after a pregnancy loss.** You may find you're withdrawn, angry, can't sleep or concentrate, are ruminating on and researching miscarriage and other health concerns. You may also experience flashbacks, a sense of numbness, irritability and distress at anything that reminds you of your loss. Up to 30 per cent of women will meet the criteria for PTSD at three months post-miscarriage. If your symptoms persist and start controlling your life, seek professional help. Asking for help is a sign of enormous courage.

❋ **Allow yourself to express all of your emotions,** whether that involves talking with loved ones or your partner, or journaling. Don't be afraid to be vulnerable with your partner, so that they can offer their support and you can heal together. Try not to blame one another for the loss.

❋ **Grief can often trigger the pain of previous traumas.** See Chapter 5 for tips on how you can help yourself in this. Having a therapist alongside you in this can be invaluable and often necessary.

Remember that no feeling is ever final, and while time doesn't necessarily heal all wounds, it will transform them. Although nobody would wish for infertility or baby loss, when we endure pain and sorrow, then our capacity to feel, to love and to tap into virtues that we never realized we had expands. We build resilience and wisdom from post-traumatic growth. In time, you can transform emotional pain into something that brings compassion and heals others, while being a source of tremendous personal power and courage. Elizabeth Day, author and broadcaster, wrote the following on social media for Mother's Day 2022: 'You are a warrior. And, one day, you will discover that your battle is also a blessing. Your wait becomes wisdom. Your pain distils into love. Your sadness transmutes itself into strength. And you then realize: these are the attributes of motherhood. What a gift that will be to your child when they come.'

When it feels right, you will be able to commemorate the loss of your baby, whether that's a ritual with your partner to honour this significant event or with your wider family. Some poignant things to do are: create a memory box, plant a tree or donate to a foundation that supports those facing baby loss (some of these wonderful charities are listed at the end of the chapter).

TCP and possible miscarriage causes

If you have had one early (first-trimester) miscarriage, in the absence of any predisposing condition, it's around 50 per cent likely to have been due to a chromosomal abnormality. It doesn't (usually) mean there is a chromosomal problem with you or your partner. Chromosomal abnormalities are when the embryo has the wrong number of chromosomes or there are structural problems with those chromosomes. Some of these embryos might self-abort very early, and a proportion might be affected by congenital abnormalities.

Chromosomal abnormalities are not necessarily due to a problem with the DNA itself. More often than not, chromosomal errors occur spontaneously during cell division after fertilization or are to do with the splitting and division as the early embryo forms. At the moment, the common medical understanding is that these errors are random events. But it's now increasingly being recognized that the epigenome potentially may control some of them. We know that the older you are, the more likely these events are. But there is research to suggest that we might be able to stabilize the chromosomes of older eggs (and older sperm), by changing their epigenetic environment via lifestyle. The same may be true for sperm quality too. For example, we know that older fathers are more likely to have babies with Klinefelter syndrome. As sperm turn over every three months, there is a real opportunity to help reduce the risk of chromosomal mishaps.

There is also likely to be an epigenetic element to those lost pregnancies that do have the correct constitution of chromosomes. Around 45 per cent of genetically normal embryos don't implant; it appears that the lining of the womb, and the cross-talk between it and the embryo, regulates whether certain genes favouring implantation will be switched on or off. The epigenome can also affect egg or sperm abnormalities. Researchers have found that compared to men who fathered chromosomally normal children, 48 per cent of sperm from the fathers of miscarried foetuses were abnormal, with sperm counts being on average 25 per cent lower. And DNA fragmentation is also higher in the sperm of men whose partners have suffered from recurrent pregnancy loss (RPL).

Recently researchers in the Netherlands observed embryos developing in the womb by using state-of-the-art imaging to create holograms of them. In the first ten weeks of development, embryos of pregnancies that ended in a miscarriage took four days longer to grow, suggesting that miscarriage may in part be the result of an embryo's growth not being quite synchronized with the growth of the tissue around it that supports its development. And research has also discovered mutations in mitochondrial DNA, especially in women with recurrent miscarriages. (There's more on the importance of mitochondrial DNA in Chapter 5.)

Some of the epigenetic mechanisms that lead to these genetic problems may be influenced by environmental factors, such as diet, toxins, exercise and even the chemical imprints of thought patterns, as described in the first part of the book. Recent evidence suggests there may be key genes, turned on or off by epi markers, that are crucial for giving the right biological instructions at each stage of foetal development. For example, Japanese scientists have recently discovered a gene in mice that needs to be suppressed for a healthy pregnancy.

There may be some spontaneous events that cannot be epigenetically controlled; some miscarriages may not be preventable. But by committing to a healthier way of living and creating a healthier epigenome, you may be able to help mitigate that risk.

Looking into recurrent pregnancy loss (RPL)

RPL is now defined as two or more first-trimester miscarriages, with new guidance now recommending investigations after experiencing two, and not three, miscarriages, as was previously the case. Testing after two can often provide enormous comfort because investigations can reveal one or more correctable factors – and it only seems right emotionally too. One of the worst aspects of recurrent miscarriage is the loss of control when you can't access the necessary investigations and solutions.

However, there may, at first, appear to be no obvious cause for RPL. This section covers a lot of possible things that go wrong, and many of these won't be covered by regular hospital investigations. Treatment, which can be medical or surgical, will depend on what tests find out – including whether you have an underlying condition. Before taking any medication or treatment, make sure you are properly counselled by your doctor. What is important for you to know is that TCP may be able to help with some of the causes of RPL and support you through the process of trying again.

A higher number of miscarriages makes it more likely that the embryos that miscarry are chromosomally normal. And having a chromosomally normal miscarriage increases the chances of a subsequent miscarriage, which is why it's important to have proper investigations to identify possible contributing factors and have time to correct them, as well as to reflect.

There's growing research to suggest that RPL can be due to epigenetic factors that affect implantation, including problems with: the embryo attaching to the womb lining, the embryo developing properly, the formation of new blood vessels, remodelling of the womb lining and progesterone levels.

As an example, one of the main epigenetic tools that controls gene behaviour is called methylation. In turn, methylation is controlled by the MTHFR gene. If there are mutations in this gene (5 per cent of people have a double mutation, and up to 60 per cent of Caucasian people have a single one), then you won't process folate correctly, increasing the risk of neural-tube defects (which is why I recommend taking methylated folate rather than folic acid – see page 90). You'll also have a high risk of raised homocysteine levels, which can affect foetal growth and increase the risk of miscarriage. You can improve methylation patterns and reduce the risk of all these consequences using lifestyle measures.

Following the pillars of TCP can positively influence your epigenetic wiring, because TCP changes the cell environment. And by doing this, it can potentially influence how the genes in the embryo behave.

Immunity, autoimmunity and hormones

The epigenome is intertwined with immunity, autoimmunity and hormonal issues involved in RPL, and there's often an interaction between all of them. In order not to reject an embryo which is genetically half foreign during implantation, the female body has to change its usual immune response. If this doesn't happen correctly, this can lead to an increased chance of the body rejecting a genetically normal embryo.

TCP will help create an epigenetic environment that can reduce the chance of genes involved in autoimmunity turning on. RPL due to immune dysregulation may be more common in women with a personal or family history of autoimmunity, blood-clotting disorders or thyroid issues (although these can sometimes be silent), as well as an environment that favours oestrogen dominance (see page 110).

One of the most common tests is for antiphospholipid and antinuclear antibodies – antibodies to the cell membrane and cell nucleus respectively. There is a whole list of other immune factors that are believed by various experts to be involved: TNF alpha, natural killer cells (NK cells) and various cytokines. You can even develop antibodies to serotonin, where the symptoms may include anxiety and depression; and to sperm (common post-vasectomy); as well as to your own hormones, including oestrogen, progesterone and human chorionic gonadotrophin (hCG is a protein made by the placenta that peaks at the end of the first trimester). Autoimmunity can increase sensitivity to stress, and as we saw in Chapter 8, this in itself can drive up inflammation and affect fertility.

A number of conditions where hormones are disturbed have been identified as possible contributors to RPL. PCOS is the most common; miscarriage can affect up to 40 per cent of women with PCOS. Others include obesity, type-2 diabetes and luteal-phase defects (a shortened cycle: see page 159), which all lead to hormonal and/or immune disturbances that can increase the chance of miscarriage. Structural issues that may affect RPL include having an irregularly-shaped uterus (such as a bicornuate uterus with two sides), and fibroids or polyps that encroach on the cavity of the uterus. Finally there's infection too, such as STDs, but also mycoplasma, toxoplasmosis (from cat faeces and undercooked meat) and others, including food poisoning through salmonella and listeria.

New studies have also found that changes to a mother's vaginal microbiome may be associated with pregnancy loss, which may be caused by bacterial imbalances. In one study, more than 50 per cent of the women who miscarried had chromosomally normal embryos and also had a reduction in the species of lactobacilli (friendly bacteria) in their vagina, and an increase in unhelpful bacteria. A diet rich in sugar, as well as exposure to chlorinated swimming pools, certain lubricants and vaginal douches, plus oral contraceptive pills and antibiotics can all upset the vaginal microbiome and throw it off-balance. An imbalance in the vaginal microbiome can be improved through nutrition, by reducing environmental toxins and by managing stress.

Many women with RPL also report generalized health issues, including pain across the body. We now know that physical symptoms can develop as a result of thoughts and trauma (see Chapters 2 and 5). And that physical pain can often be a sign of unresolved and unprocessed emotion and trauma in the body. Treating the emotional as well as physical components of well-being really matters and should always be done together. This is what you can invest in, to give your next pregnancy the best chance possible.

TESTS YOU MAY BE OFFERED FOR RPL

After two (or three) miscarriages, tests include an ultrasound scan to assess if there are any structural issues or any masses that may be an issue; an STD screen to check for common infections; a saline sonogram, or HSG (hysterosalpingogram) or HyCoSy, to assess the uterine cavity and Fallopian tubes; an endometrial biopsy to assess the uterine lining for hormonal problems, luteal-phase defects (see page 159) or inflammation; and a hysteroscopy that involves looking into the uterine cavity with a camera to assess any scarring, masses or structural abnormalities and to treat them. Blood tests include looking at hormone levels, antibodies, bacterial and viral screens, thyroid function, diabetes, clotting factors, chromosomal testing (karyotyping) of the couple, and chromosomal testing of the baby and/or placenta.

Additional tests can be done to assess various gene mutations and potential immune causes, but these are not necessarily recognized or encouraged. They are carried out in some specialist centres and should be interpreted by someone with experience and understanding of treatment in this field.

When is it safe to try again?

This is the question that most people ask following a miscarriage. If you've had one miscarriage the answer is: don't rush into it. You're ready when you feel emotionally and physically prepared. Take time to process your trauma and grief, individually and/or as a couple. I often advise patients to wait at least until they've had one normal menstrual cycle, to help the body rebalance. If you have only just started TCP, ideally you'll do it for three months (or more) before trying again.

If you've had more than one consecutive miscarriage, you need time for investigations as well as to optimize your body and mind. How long you will wait will depend on your personal circumstances, not least your age, but it's important to adjust and correct any contributing factors. Remember, the time you spend investing in yourself and healing is time that will count towards improving your chances of conceiving, carrying to term and having the healthiest possible child.

The emotional underside of pregnancy loss

Given that early pregnancy is governed by hormonal, immune and biochemical processes that can be affected by the mind, it's worth looking at the emotional patterns that can be connected to miscarriage.

Women with a history of psychological stress, or those who have had recent negative life events, appear to be twice as likely to have a chromosomally normal miscarriage. Doctors are often keen to dispel any concerns over stress having an impact on pregnancy, but reflecting what the research shows is not the same as blaming women.

Issues that contribute to stress may include emotional trauma, social problems, financial concerns, partnership disharmony, changes in personal circumstances, work pressure and, ironically, previous pregnancy loss. There will of course always be unavoidable life events and circumstances, which makes it even more vital that our healthcare systems get better at managing mental and emotional health, and our societies need to start enforcing supportive employment practices for women and men experiencing trauma and stress, including miscarriage.

Interestingly, when questioned, 76 per cent of women feel that negative stress can affect pregnancy outcomes and, in my experience, women's instincts tend to be correct. If this is you, although you can't change any difficult life events you may be experiencing, hopefully finding some support will help you deal with its impact and the way you can manage your stress, even transforming it into something positive.

CASE STUDY

One of my patients, Ella, aged forty-three, had a partner who was a musician, who often worked abroad. She found this stressful because frequently he wasn't home around the time of ovulation. Ella had a first-trimester miscarriage, then one unsuccessful round of IVF. She developed anger and resentment towards her partner, blaming him for the baby loss and infertility that she was left to manage on her own.

When she started therapy, Ella came to realize that she was in an old pattern of abandonment that was influencing her life decisions and contributing to significant stress, which had started with her father, who left home early in her life and was rarely around. From then on, Ella felt responsible for protecting and looking after her mother, often at the neglect of her own emotional needs. Relationships with unavailable men perpetuated this wound, which stemmed from being abandoned early in life, which she had not healed. Eventually Ella separated from her partner, deciding that she wanted to become a single mother, and took time to heal with the help of a counsellor. The unprocessed trauma from her father's abandonment was something she realized had been affecting her and contributing to her trajectory, so healing this was an important step in cultivating a sense of safety in her body, in preparation for pregnancy.

It's worth exploring any possible trauma or emotional discord; research shows that having psychotherapy appears to significantly improve the chance of carrying a pregnancy to full term. These are other possible emotional patterns that you may find yourself relating to:

- ❊ Despite wanting a child, you may have mixed feelings that you can't express. You may feel your partner wants to have a child more than you do. Or the only way to gain recognition as a woman is by becoming a mother. Or that becoming a mother is what's expected of you. Or you might feel a loss of control over your body or being pushed into the decision.

- ❊ You may know that having a baby could create conflict in, or impose difficulties on, your relationship. This may be due to unspoken differences about parenthood between you and your partner.

- ❊ If you had a difficult childhood, you may have doubts about your ability to be a good parent and have an unspoken need to protect any child from having the same experience.

- ❊ You may have feelings of being trapped in a situation, or not being able to exert a choice or influence over your body. The same may be true of other parts of your life: a feeling of loss of control and being pushed into decisions.

If you find yourself resonating with any of the above, or dealing with baby loss, it can be really helpful to seek the assistance of a counsellor in order to work through these issues.

TCP to recover from miscarriage or baby loss

TCP can be used to help you recover from a miscarriage, both physically and emotionally, while giving your body the best chance of carrying your next pregnancy. You can also customize TCP by adding in the following:

Nutrition

* **Eat foods rich in iron to compensate for blood loss**: these include meat, shellfish, leafy greens, beans, brown rice, dark chocolate and pumpkin seeds. You may need to take an iron supplement, which can cause constipation, so eat good amounts of fibre and drink plenty of liquids. Supplement with vitamin C and eat vitamin C-rich foods, such as citrus and strawberries, to help iron absorption.

* **Magnesium-rich foods can help with depression, anxiety and mood disturbances**: these include beans, nuts and dark chocolate.

* **Try to avoid comfort-eating low-GI foods**, such as instant rice, noodles, sugary foods and baked goods, although this can be hard when you're feeling low. They can cause your blood-sugar levels to swing, which fuels inflammation.

* **Eat lots of protein to help you to heal and recover**: fish, eggs, lentils, grains, quinoa and lean meat.

* **Support your thyroid function by eating seaweed.**

* **Consider getting tested for dairy, wheat and gluten intolerance** if you suffer from bloating, excessive tiredness, headaches, irritability, frequent changes of bowel habit or gut pain. Or adjust your diet to eliminate them for a short

period and see how you feel. Coeliac disease has been associated with recurrent miscarriage as well as infertility and menstrual abnormalities.

* **Drink raspberry-leaf and nettle tea**, which can help to ease muscle spasm, cramping and pain, aiding the uterus to return to normal.

* **Avoid comfort-eating low-fibre carbs**, such as instant rice, noodles and pretzels, which can cause significant swings in your blood-sugar levels and contribute to inflammation.

* **Avoid soft cheese, unpasteurized dairy products and raw meat** – don't consume food that can provide a breeding ground for bacteria, in order to avoid infection.

* **Avoid soya-based products**, as they can prevent you absorbing enough iron.

* **Consume lots of fluid in the form of filtered water, coconut water and pure (unsweetened) orange juice** to help iron absorption.

* **Eat foods that contain folate**, such as spinach, kale, broccoli, nuts and seeds.

* **Take methylated folate**, as the prevalence of the MTHFR mutation is high.

* **If you've spent a long time on hormonal contraception**, you may need to boost your levels of various vitamins and minerals (see Chapter 17).

* **Consider a chlorophyll supplement** to help regulate the immune system.

Exercise

Exercise can maintain good blood flow to the pelvic organs, as well as being beneficial for mental health. But go very gently if you're experiencing any physical symptoms, including bleeding and pain, and also early pregnancy symptoms, such as headaches and tiredness. Stick to gentle walking and yoga, listen to your body and don't push yourself. Build up gradually to 150 minutes a week.

Stress

* **Miscarriage may bring a deep need for spiritual connection**: many people find holistic treatments helpful in processing unintegrated trauma and in dealing with stress. Acupuncture can help to restore blood flow and chi (energy) to the reproductive organs. Shamanic healing can help you reconnect with lost parts of yourself, and with your baby. Reiki can help to restore energetic flow and clear impediments and emotional trauma. Aromatherapy can help with stored tension and anxieties. Osteopathy and chiropractic can relieve tension in your muscles, helping to restore the natural realignment of the pelvic organs. Energetic healing can get you back into balance so that you can process grief through your body.

* **If words are hard to find to express your emotions,** you can do this through art. And creating something may give your experience a solid, physical form.

* **Soak in soothing herbal baths:** you can add yarrow, lavender, sage, rosemary and Epsom salts for stress relief and their antibacterial effects. However, avoid bathing if you're still bleeding and wearing tampons at this time, to reduce the risk of infection.

* **When you meditate,** hold gratitude for yourself and all that your incredible body has gone through.

Some notes for partners

In baby loss, partners are often overlooked, even though you will feel grief, sadness, confusion and anger too. If you are a man, you may be interested to know that 73 per cent of men going through miscarriage say they have felt they had to 'stay strong'. This belief is tied into the culturally reinforced, toxic idea that expressing emotion somehow makes you less of a man. It can lead to around 10 per cent of men developing PTSD following the loss. Around the same number feel that even if they do want to talk, there isn't enough support available. But talking is one of the most important things you can do:

* **Acknowledge the physicality and emotional intensity of your partner's loss**, as her body has gone through it. Keep talking and offer support, whether it's being there to hold her or offer words of comfort. You may find that you shift into problem-solving mode when you see your partner in distress. Rather than focusing on fixing, share how you're feeling and help her to feel safe in doing the same.

* **Don't rush through grief**: if you both need to spend time at home together, give yourself permission to take time off work.

* **Don't blame yourself for the loss**, as many partners do. It can lead you into a negative emotional spiral.

* **Having sex may take some time**, as it may be emotionally triggering and possibly painful. Go gradually, keep communicating and give each other space, when needed.

* **Look after yourself and your feelings**: seeing a counsellor together to deal with your grief and any relationship strains can be incredibly beneficial and can help you to heal and process. Using holistic therapies may also be very helpful for processing emotions.

* **You can only support your partner if you also take care of yourself**: you can share your experience and feelings with your friends, but it may also be helpful to find a forum where there are other men who have been through baby

loss. Consider keeping a journal to express your feelings, if you find them difficult to articulate.

✻ **Start a project or something you can do with your partner**: finding an outlet where you can both experience adventure and happiness may help you tap into who you were before the loss.

✻ **Know that you may react and cope differently from your partner**: this is normal. Try not to judge one another, but to be compassionate towards each other. Remember that so much of your previous life experience as individuals can condition how you feel and respond in adversity, so be respectful of the other's views and feelings.

Further support

There are lots of helpful organizations to assist you through this difficult time. Here are just a few suggestions:

✻ ARC (Antenatal Results and Choices): www.arc-uk.org

✻ Dad Pad: www.thedadpad.co.uk/

✻ Ectopic Pregnancy Foundation: www.ectopicpregnancy. co.uk

✻ Ectopic Pregnancy Trust: www.ectopic.org.uk

✻ Kicks Count: www.kickscount.org.uk

✻ Life After Loss: www.lifeafterloss.org.uk

✻ Lullaby Trust: www.lullabytrust.org.uk

✻ Mariposa Trust: www.mariposatrust.org/

✻ Miscarriage Association: www.miscarriageassociation. org.uk/

❋ Miscarriage for Men: www.miscarriageformen.com/

❋ Sands: www.sands.org.uk

❋ Tommy's: www.tommys.org

❋ Twins Trust: www.twinstrust.org

CHAPTER 13

TCP for fertility after thirty-five

You'll have heard that female fertility goes into a steep decline after the age of thirty-five. But do you also know that the only age group where babies are on the increase is among women aged forty and over? In the UK the number of babies born to women aged fifty and over has quadrupled over the past twenty years, to more than 200 a year.

Later motherhood is now a fact of life. I want to enable women to optimize their health and to conceive when it's right for them. Quite often this may be later in life. It's entirely possible to look after and continue to enhance your fertility into your forties, despite what you may be told. Indeed there is a lot of good news when it comes to being a parent later in life. You may already have some significant advantages over younger parents: solid finances, wisdom that comes with experience, and possibly the ability to spend more time with your children, if you have achieved certain career milestones. There is some data to suggest that children born to later-life parents seem to have a higher-than-average IQ and better academic performance. The life expectancy of older parents also appears to be higher, with a greater overall chance of reaching the age of ninety-five. And they seem to be better protected against dementia and cognitive decline.

But perhaps most importantly of all, older-age parents bring a different consciousness to the process of conceiving. Despite the fact that, for some, this may have been a consequence of various curveballs experienced during life, for others it's a conscious decision to postpone childbearing until a certain level of self-evolution and accomplishment has been achieved. This is almost always an active decision and reflects a deep commitment to the role of parenthood and its responsibilities. It also often means that the potential parent has reached a certain level of healing that comes with age, enabling them to step into the fullness of responsibility and requirements that come with being a parent.

Age and fertility

Women are born with around two million eggs. By the age of puberty, this number reduces to between 300,000 and 500,000. Around age thirty-five the decline speeds up, so that by about thirty-seven the number is down to 25,000. And by the age of fifty-one, it's 1,000. When it comes to egg quality, over time the DNA of eggs can gradually become damaged. This is a key reason (along with declining sperm quality and changes in your reproductive health) for the rise in miscarriage rates with age too. Between thirty-five and forty-five, 20–35 per cent of pregnancies end this way, and over the age of forty-five, it's 50 per cent.

Alongside egg quality and quantity declining during your forties, there are significant changes in your hormones too, causing cycles to become erratic and marking the beginning of the perimenopause (see page 245). And age also increases the chance of developing gynaecological conditions that can interfere with fertility, such as endometriosis, fibroids and polyps (see Chapter 16).

Sadly, IVF is not a cure for age; success rates over the age of forty – in particular in terms of live births – are not much better than natural conception rates. IVF cannot improve egg quality and is limited by the number of eggs available. For women aged forty to forty-two, average IVF success rates are 11 per cent; for women aged forty-three to forty-four, this reduces to 5 per cent; and for women over the age of forty-four, it goes down to 4 per cent and lower.

Age can also bring a higher chance of miscarriage, congenital abnormalities and complications such as pre-eclampsia, diabetes, preterm birth and operative assistance at birth. There is also a rise in chromosomal abnormalities in embryos, which can lead to, for example, Down's syndrome. Historical and patriarchal views of motherhood label women over thirty-five as 'geriatric' mothers. Yet, ironically, there's no equivalent phrase to describe the fact that male age affects conception and the health of the baby too. Regardless of female age, having a male partner over the age of forty gives a 30 per cent lower chance of conception over a year than having a partner who's less than thirty years old. (If you're a man, see Chapter 11 for advice on age and fertility.)

How do you know how fertile you are?

The usual way to measure ovarian reserve is by scanning the ovaries – to count the follicles – plus a blood test measuring anti-Müllerian hormone (AMH), a hormone produced by the ovaries; and sometimes also FSH, a hormone produced by the brain.

However, a recent study has shown that levels of these two hormones don't accurately correlate with a woman's future fertility. The study looked at women between the ages of thirty and forty-four and found that those whose hormonal markers seemed to show diminished ovarian reserve (an AMH below 0.7 or an FSH of 10 or more) did not have a statistically lower risk of having a live birth, compared to women with normal markers. This means that even if you've been told your blood tests are showing low ovarian reserve, you do have the potential to conceive with your own eggs. It's also more evidence that the epigenetic environment of the eggs is the key factor driving conception rates, rather than genetics.

CASE STUDY

For example, I met Calista when she was forty-two years old. She was dealing with several past traumas and a series of dysregulated relationships. After having counselling, she felt herself to be ready to become a mother on her own. However, her AMH was very low, at 0.2. Most doctors would have considered this reason enough to use donor eggs, but Calista really wanted to attempt it with her own eggs first. We discussed ways in which she could improve her diet, as well as exercise and how to manage her stress. And after one round of mild (low-dose stimulation) IVF, along with sperm donation from a regulated donor, she became pregnant.

There is an important clue that you may be missing if you're finding it hard to get pregnant at a later age. When I ask questions about a patient's reproductive past, it often becomes clear that she has been sexually active for a long time, hasn't always used contraception, but has never got pregnant. Up to 45 per cent of pregnancies are unplanned; if someone is having enough sex and not being meticulous about contraception, the chances are they will become pregnant. And so it seems likely that even when younger, some of these patients' fertility may have been low. In other words, what's labelled as 'older-age infertility' may sometimes be younger-age subfertility that was never investigated. This is why being aware of your fertility from a younger age is so important, and taking an interest in preserving and caring for it is key.

Protecting your egg reserves

By doing TCP, you can help shift the odds in favour not only of conception, but also towards reducing the chances of miscarriage and improving the chances of having a healthy child. This goes back to the egg. Keeping your eggs well nourished is important at any age, but if you're over thirty-five it's the single most important thing you can do. The human egg is a cell that's both unusual and amazing – when activated, it can create a whole human being – and it's the biggest cell in the body. It stops halfway through its growth and stays in suspended animation in the ovary, for several decades, until it begins the process leading towards ovulation. How well the egg is able to hold its DNA in a stable configuration during this time in storage determines to a large extent whether it will fertilize and give rise to a healthy child.

A handful of eggs come out of storage three months before one is released by ovulation, although the initial recruitment occurs around a year before ovulation. Research has shown that follicular fluid surrounding the egg at this time has a key epigenetic role and influences egg quality. So the year, and in particular the three months, leading up to when you plan to start trying is when the lifestyle choices you make are specially important and can impact on the quality of the egg.

An egg contains DNA in its nucleus and has a membrane like other cells, but on top of the membrane it also has a coating called the zona pellucida, which communicates with both the follicle and sperm and acts a bit like a second cell membrane. Inside the egg, the nucleus is surrounded by cytoplasm, which contains the epi markers that control its genes. (In fact cytoplasm is so much in control that when transplanted to a different kind of cell entirely, it can create the beginnings of a baby; this is how Dolly the sheep was cloned!) The cytoplasm is under the influence of the cell membrane, which (as you learned in Chapter 1) is like the brain of the cell. So even before the DNA in the egg gets to act, there's the zona pellucida, cell membrane and cytoplasm that control what happens. Anything influencing the follicles (all the factors discussed in this book) will also influence the growth and development of the egg cell.

While the number of eggs that you start with is largely predestined by genetics, and while you cannot stop egg numbers dropping as you age, you can improve the egg's environment and leverage the power of epigenetics to counter DNA damage and protect your egg quality. Doing this may also reduce the rate at which egg numbers decline.

Studies suggest that the decline of ovarian function is linked to the shortening of telomeres (the caps on DNA that get smaller with ageing). And we know that diet, exercise, stress management and social support can reduce the rate of this decline by increasing the concentration of telomerase, the enzyme that helps preserve telomeres, and so potentially it may even change the rate of ovarian and egg ageing. A study in mice showed that supplementing their diet with antioxidants, such as coenzyme Q10, kept their eggs in better shape, along with improving mitochondrial function, which contributed to better live birth rates.

CASE STUDY

Hailey had always wanted to become a mother. But she had a fear of giving birth, in part because her mother had lost a baby at twenty weeks of pregnancy. Hailey had often engaged in unprotected sex with previous long-term partners, but had never conceived. She knew there was some healing to do and joined a women's healing group, where the focus was on connecting deeply with the body using sound, meditation, movement and energy work.

She found, when she connected with her womb, that she felt a lot of grief and trauma that was stored there. Some of this was to do with relationships Hailey had had with men who were emotionally unavailable, but she also identified that the grief was associated with disempowerment, manipulation, abandonment and suppression that affected the maternal ancestral line. The journey of healing went on for a few years, as she continued to excavate and process the full extent of previously repressed emotions, experienced by generations of women in her family, learning to attend to her own emotional needs.

When she was forty-five Hailey met the man she knew would be the father of her child. She told me that most of her friends thought she was in a fantasy world and, although medically the statistics were not on her side, she felt a deep sense that pregnancy was still possible. Sure enough, when she was forty-six and a half, she fell pregnant naturally.

Then, at twenty weeks of pregnancy, she began to have cramps. After a scan, it became clear that her cervix was starting to open, drawing similarities to her mother's experience. But Hailey had a strong sense that her baby was here to stay. She did a lot of work to clear the ancestral trauma that she still felt she was holding in the cervical area, along with the Mother Wound, and followed the medical advice given to her to rest. After five weeks her cervix had stabilized and she was discharged from hospital. She went into labour at thirty-seven weeks and gave birth to a beautiful and healthy baby girl.

GOING SOLO

More women are taking control of their destiny by choosing to have children on their own, often later in life, through sperm donation or co-parenting with friends. Women are also freezing their eggs or embryos, for use later in life. Mel Johnson, of The Stork and I, decided to go it alone when she didn't meet the right partner at the right time. 'It took me a long time to make the decision to take this path, mainly because I needed to work through letting go of the fairy-tale way I had expected to become a parent. At thirty-eight, following IVF with donor sperm, I had my daughter. If I would have known how amazing being a solo parent would be, I would have worried about it much less and started the process sooner.'

A lot of research has now shown that solo mothers are more than capable of providing a positive and secure upbringing for their children, and tend to be well prepared before becoming a parent. Their children have been described as having fewer emotional and behavioural difficulties compared to children from mothers in relationships. Yet single women continue to be discriminated against and stigmatized; for example, they can't access free assisted reproductive technologies on the NHS. Everybody needs better access to affordable fertility treatment, including single mothers.

Menopause and fertility

For most women the menopause starts in their forties, and can last from several months up to ten years. Some of the first signs of the perimenopause are a change in menstrual pattern to irregular or sporadic bleeding, changes in mood, hot flashes, tiredness, joint aches and pains, alterations in the skin, hair loss, sex becoming more painful, night sweats, trouble concentrating, brain fog, an increase in urinary-tract infections (UTIs), vaginal dryness and pain and increased anxiety.

Menopause marks the end of egg reserves, but it's clinically defined as periods having stopped for a full year. In the UK the average age is between forty-eight and fifty-two, although it can be earlier or later.

If menopause happens before the age of forty-five it's called an early menopause. If your mother had early menopause, your chances increase too (though it doesn't make it inevitable). Early menopause may also be due to a medical condition, illness or surgery. Before forty, it's called premature menopause or premature ovarian insufficiency (POI). This affects around 1 per cent of women and can be due to genetic conditions, such as Turner syndrome (the absence of an X chromosome) and Fragile X syndrome (where the X chromosomes are easily damaged). Around 10 per cent of women with premature menopause can get pregnant naturally, but as cycles (and therefore ovulation) may be erratic, it can be difficult and highly unpredictable. Where egg reserves are extremely low or if you're in the menopause and haven't previously frozen eggs or embryos (see Chapter 14), your remaining option for carrying a child is egg donation (see also Chapter 14).

CASE STUDY

One of my patients, Rosie, became perimenopausal at the age of thirty-five. She had a traumatic birth, as she was born preterm and was immediately separated from her mother to go into neonatal care. Later on she developed several autoimmune conditions and allergies, as well as a throat tic. An issue in the jaw area can mean there are difficulties expressing and articulating your truth (see page 195 in the 12-week plan on how the jaw and pelvis are closely interlinked). Rosie's parents divorced when she was very young. She grew up surrounded by conflict, internalizing a lot of guilt and shouldering too many responsibilities. As an adult, she described herself as 'dysregulated' and 'constantly wired'. By the time she came to see me, she'd had several rounds of IVF, without success. This had only added to her stress.

When we met, I spent time getting Rosie to tune into her emotions and where they were in her body. She started feeling a pain in her stomach and told me this was where she'd often experienced bloating after getting upset. It felt to her like resentment. And when she sat with it, she found it rising into her throat, making her feel she was suffocating. This whole process – of getting her to encounter, recognize and hold space for her emotions – led Rosie to realize that she had a visceral fear of death, having come so close to it as a baby. And she also recognized that her fear extended to pregnancy.

Rosie may try again with her own eggs or she may use donor eggs. What is important for conception is that she addressed the emotional aspects of her infertility, and that her body and mind now feel safe and regulated. The trauma that Rosie experienced set the scene for her premature ovarian ageing, and we now have research that shows a correlation between earlier-life trauma and reduced ovarian reserve later in life (see Chapter 5), but this doesn't mean that it will continue to prevent her from conceiving.

TCP advice for aged over thirty-five

TCP advice in the pillars chapters (Chapters 6–10) and the 12-week plan (see pages 145–200) is relevant for any age, but with increasing age it becomes even more important to follow it. Each TCP pillar is key to improving the environment of the egg (and sperm), and can positively impact on their quality and on your overall natural fertility.

CHAPTER 14

TCP for assisted reproductive technologies (including IVF)

Sometimes people need medical assistance to conceive. There's no denying that IVF is an incredible technology: it's responsible for the births of more than eight million babies around the world, helping create families that wouldn't otherwise have existed, and enhancing the lives of millions of people.

However, IVF and other assisted reproductive technologies (ARTs) are not a cure for infertility (see page 52). IVF was originally invented to bypass Fallopian-tube issues, and it's still often the only way to conceive when someone has Fallopian tubes that are blocked, damaged or absent. But the use of IVF has broadened considerably over the last several decades, when it's become necessary in other situations too: egg-freezing and embryo-freezing, single women, same-sex couples, surrogacy and as part of fertility preservation treatment for transgender people and those undergoing cancer treatment. It can also be helpful when conception is taking a long time (and you feel you're running out of time), and for reduced ovarian reserve, male infertility, medical conditions that can make conception more difficult and to avoid specific genetic abnormalities that may have been identified.

The problem is that ART is often recommended before there has been a proper chance to assess or improve someone's natural fertility. And ART is frequently suggested to people who are diagnosed with unexplained infertility, where more detailed questioning and investigations might reveal several 'explained' issues that are contributing to the problem. Before going down the route of ART, it's important to look at any underlying condition or contributing factors, as described in the first part of this book. ART – whether it is IVF or intrauterine insemination (IUI) – will not make you more fertile; it is simply a way of helping bring together eggs and sperm and encouraging implantation. In addition, the latest research is showing that it can take on average a total of three full IVF cycles to achieve a live birth, meaning that most people will need more than one IVF cycle, regardless of age, and that each cycle may involve several embryo transfers. Even in younger age groups, the success of IVF in a first round is often no more than 50 per cent, and this only improves up to a certain point following another one or two rounds, after which a ceiling appears to be reached.

My advice, if you're needing this kind of assistance after a full exploration of any contributing issues, is to do TCP before having ART, and then alongside it too. This applies if you're in a couple, but also if you're single and are having your eggs or sperm frozen; or if you're in a same-sex relationship acting as the donor or carrier. The investment you're making in your body, your eggs and your sperm is one that will naturally improve your ability to conceive and carry a pregnancy, as well as your long-term health and your child's too. At the outset, ART may appear to have all the answers, but unless contributing factors are addressed first, they may continue to affect you later in life and potentially influence the health of any children you have.

Are you ready to have assisted conception (ART)?

The answer to this is totally individual. Generally speaking, many people are either encouraged to start ART too soon or are given very few other options. When treatment wasn't as readily available during the pandemic, many couples found that they conceived naturally. And a US study using data from European cities, including London, found that in women aged thirty-five to thirty-nine, fewer than one in ten failed to conceive naturally after two years, unless the male partner was over forty.

Some women I treat in their early forties will go straight to ART after trying for six months, and others will try naturally for a year or for two. Trying naturally and doing TCP is a good option if there aren't any major obstacles to getting pregnant, such as a health condition, gynaecological disorder or very low ovarian reserve. But even then, continuing to try naturally may still be possible, because TCP will benefit various coexisting conditions, such as endometriosis or PCOS, and will help to look after your eggs and sperm. How long for is different for everyone and depends on individual circumstances. If you've been trying for a period of time without success, it's important to get tested, as you need to know about any obstacles (see page 50 for tests) and have a discussion with a supportive doctor, who can help to guide you and provide a wider perspective on your options. It's also vital to discuss what you wish to do as a couple (or with your personal support network, if you're conceiving as a single mother). Knowledge will empower you to make the right decision for you. And remember: only you can decide on what's best for you.

How do you choose a clinic?

Assuming that you are ready to go ahead with ART, you may first have to consider geography, NHS funding and/or price. But if you do have a choice of clinics, don't base your decision solely on success rates. Remember, clinics can present this data in different formats, such as reporting on pregnancy rates instead of babies born, and they are free to select the categories of patients they treat. If you are interested in success rates, the best place to look is the Human Fertilisation & Embryology Authority (HFEA) website, as it standardizes how these rates are reported. You'll see that the variation between clinics is small.

There are other factors that I'd argue are more important, namely if the clinic and their approach is a good fit for you. How accessible is the clinic to you? Do you align with the clinic's values? Do you like their approach to treatment? What is the rationale behind their treatment protocol? Do the staff seem encouraging and supportive? You can find out by going to open days or having a short consultation; many clinics offer one for free.

What are the main ART methods?

Don't jump into having the most expensive treatment with the most intervention because it has the highest reported success rate. There is often more than one option, and less intervention can often mean fewer side-effects. Below is a general rundown of possible treatments, starting with the least interventional.

Fertility medications

Ovarian stimulation drugs are for women who aren't ovulating each month or ovulate irregularly. They can also be used in the first part of IUI and IVF. Their role is to stimulate the growth of follicles and lead to the maturation of any eggs they contain. They should be used alongside monitoring via blood tests/scans, because overstimulation increases the chance of multiple births, which may be riskier, and ovarian hyperstimulation syndrome.

Medications can have side-effects, such as bloating and possibly abdominal tenderness, fluid retention, nausea, headaches, irritability and blurred vision. They also affect the environment the eggs are exposed to and can potentially influence the integrity and expression of egg DNA through their epigenetic effects. When used for prolonged periods of time, medications carry an increased risk of hormonal reproductive cancers, so it's important that their dosage and length of time used are kept to a minimum. They include Clomiphene (clomid) and Tamoxifen/letrozole as well as gonadotrophins – the injectable drugs most commonly used during IVF.

Intrauterine insemination (IUI)

Sperm from your partner or a donor is washed and concentrated, then placed via a catheter into the uterine cavity. IUI's chances of success are limited by the quality of the sperm and the environment of the Fallopian tubes. It is done either with or without fertility medication. You are also often given a shot of hCG (human chorionic gonadotrophin), the hormone that triggers ovulation.

IUI is less invasive and costly than IVF, although it has less chance of success too. It's generally reserved for under-thirty-fives in couples (sometimes up to forty), single women under forty, lesbian couples, for some cases of irregular ovulation and where there are issues with erection and/or ejaculation. Usually several attempts are needed. The pregnancy rate is around 10–15 per cent with each cycle, reaching a maximum of 20–25 per cent after four to six cycles.

IVF (in vitro fertilization)

This is the most common ART procedure and the one with the highest success rate. However, it's not a cure for infertility, as it's often mistakenly assumed to be. The success of IVF is dependent on age and all the factors explored in TCP that contribute to fertile health. IVF can improve your chances by increasing the number of eggs produced, especially over several rounds, but it can't improve egg quality; and in some cases, depending on the stimulation used, it may even have negative epigenetic effects on eggs. That is one reason why I advocate milder stimulation protocols (see below).

IVF involves ovarian stimulation with drugs, encouraging multiple follicles to grow and their eggs to develop, plus often a second drug to prevent premature ovulation and regulate growth. When there are enough follicles, a hormone called beta human chorionic gonadotrophin (beta hCG) is prescribed to start the final stage of egg maturation. Thirty-six hours later the eggs are collected by inserting a needle through the vagina and into the ovaries. At the same time fresh sperm is collected from your partner (or the frozen/donor sperm is thawed).

The sperm and collected eggs are combined in a dish in the lab for fertilization. The fertilized eggs are allowed to grow and develop for a few days, forming embryos and eventually blastocysts (a five- to six-day-old embryo). These are either transferred fresh, or are frozen and used later (or they can be donated, see below). Success depends on many factors, including age, but there is a better success rate if the eggs are from a young patient or donor. Success is cumulative over a number of cycles, but only up to a certain point, because IVF can't improve egg quality.

One key risk is ovarian hyperstimulation syndrome (OHSS), which occurs in its mild form in up to 33 per cent of women having IVF treatment. It's when too many follicles grow and the ovaries swell, leading to bloating and fluid retention as well as the release of substances that trigger widespread inflammation. It can require hospitalization and even intensive care, in its severest form. IVF also slightly increases the chance of ectopic pregnancy, as well as pre-eclampsia, low birth weight and birth defects.

Mild or natural IVF

Natural-cycle or mild IVF uses the approach of 'less is more', with lower doses of stimulation drugs (or an absence of them altogether). It has fewer side-effects, such as less risk of OHSS, is less expensive and may also yield better results and healthier babies. And the lower amount of stimulation may be all that's required for some people, whether this is a younger patient with good ovarian reserve or an older patient with lower reserves.

Mild IVF has other benefits too: it minimizes the competition for nutrients between eggs and encourages the growth of what may be better-quality eggs. It also minimizes the downsides of gonadotrophin drugs; high levels can create an adverse environment that may compromise egg DNA as well as reduce the chances of successful implantation. Natural or mild IVF may also impact less on the health of any future children than regular IVF does.

Intracytoplasmic sperm injection (ICSI)

ICSI is when, during IVF, instead of the sperm and eggs being placed together and left to fertilize, the sperm is injected into the egg. It's used when sperm has low counts, poor motility and/or an increased number of abnormalities. In the absence of severe male-factor issues, ICSI has not been shown to improve overall pregnancy rates and is often offered at additional cost on top of IVF. Some clinics do ICSI for all cases. Even if ICSI is used, it's important to give natural measures time to improve the overall quality of the sperm before the procedure, to optimize the chance of success and a healthy baby, especially as ICSI has some risks. For example, sperm used in ICSI are likely to have significantly more DNA damage, the consequences of which can be passed on to a future child. ICSI may potentially increase the chance of infertility in subsequent male offspring, can contribute to a slightly higher risk of birth defects and of possible health issues for any future child later down the line. Whether this is due to the technique itself or the fact that the sperm used in ICSI often has abnormalities, or a combination of both, remains to be determined (see Chapter 11).

Egg, sperm and embryo donation

There are still stigma and shame around embryo and sperm donation. But these are simply different versions of the unique road to parenthood. There's a whole range of different reasons as to why someone may use donor conception, and normalizing this is vital in terms of improving people's access to a family.

Eggs and sperm can be donated anonymously, or not. Eggs can be donated by an altruistic donor. This might be a woman who is having IVF (this often includes a discount on her treatment) or someone you know who agrees to be the donor. Egg donation tends to be used by women who have low ovarian reserves, whether due to age or a medical condition. It's also used by gay couples (in a lesbian couple, this donation can be from one partner to the other) and single men using a surrogate. Egg or sperm donation is also used by those who may not have undergone fertility preservation ahead of cancer treatment or gender reassignment, or where this was unsuccessful. Sperm donation is used when a single woman or a lesbian couple wishes to conceive, or when a man has no sperm, or sperm that can't fertilize. Sperm or eggs can also be frozen before gender reassignment and used at a later date. Sometimes egg and sperm donation are done to prevent genetic conditions being passed on to the child. Finally, embryo donation also happens when a woman or couple has finished having children and ART and wants to help other singles or couples who are struggling to conceive.

Some of the stigma is attributed to what's perceived as a diminished biological relationship. But in fact epigenetics plays a large part – you could argue even larger than genetics – in forming a baby. It can control genetic inheritance through the process of epigenetic switching, where certain genes are turned on and off, affecting everything from brain development and metabolism, through to immunity and hormonal health.

Children are so much more than simply the genes they carry. They are embodiments of how those genes and the surrounding environment combine to give rise to the unique individual. The resulting child of egg or sperm donation is therefore always a beautiful, unique combination of the donor and carrier. In fact a child's personality may be anywhere between 50 and 70 per cent due to experiences and environment rather than genes.

The science behind epigenetics is growing. Researchers have studied microRNA (miRNA), part of an epigenetic mechanism that's responsible for fine-tuning gene activity, including everything from growth and development to personality and immunity. MicroRNAs have been found in fluid from the womb lining during implantation. Research into one particular microRNA showed that it was incorporated into mice embryos and affected several genes in those embryos.

One big question that often arises is whether egg or sperm donation should be considered sooner than it usually is. This is most relevant to those who are older or have reduced ovarian reserve or abnormal sperm. In truth, there is no right or wrong answer. This decision needs careful and considered counselling and discussion, especially as there are implications both for the parents and for the children born through the process.

'When we made the decision to move to donor eggs, I had many fears and questions,' says Becky Kearns, founder of Paths to Parent*hub*. 'Would I ever truly feel like or be seen as a *"real"* mum? Would I bond with my child in the way I'd always imagined? Would they have some kind of sixth sense that we weren't genetically related? I've since found that these fears, although very real at the time, were completely unfounded and couldn't be further from the truth. From once feeling like the unluckiest person in the world, I now, as a mum to three incredible girls, feel so lucky that I get the privilege of being not just "a mum", but *their* mum.'

A NOTE ON SPERM DONATION

Due to a shortage of donors, some women have little choice but to use an unofficial, private donor. But this can put you at risk. It's important that a donor is screened for any potential conditions and infections that could be passed on, and that their sperm is tested too. If not screened, an unofficial donor could be unaware of any problems. And some unregulated donors are unethical: one red flag is the man asking for insemination via intercourse. There have been cases of some men fathering hundreds of children, whereas regulated donors are only allowed to donate up to ten families. Also, regulated donors legally absolve themselves of a claim on the child that's born; there is no such legal contract with unregulated donors. Even if you find a sperm donor privately, it's important that the treatment takes place in a clinical setting to minimize any risks.

Pre-implantation genetic testing (PGT)

This is when embryos made during IVF are screened for chromosomal abnormalities or specific genetic mutations. It's done either to optimize the success of IVF by choosing only genetically normal embryos, or to avoid passing on inherited genetic conditions. However, it can't screen for epigenetic information and so it's not 100 per cent reliable. And sometimes the genetic result isn't clear-cut, but there's a risk that further testing might compromise the embryo. Sometimes all the embryos may have abnormalities, in which case there may be no embryo to transfer. Testing at such an early stage may not even give a totally reliable result. Pregnancy is far more complicated than genetics alone, as this book has shown, and therefore PGT is a field where more research is needed; in the absence of screening for specific genetic disorders, experts have yet to reach a consensus on how useful it is.

Egg-freezing

Egg-freezing has become increasingly popular – the number of treatments doubled in 2020 compared to the previous year. The treatment is the same as IVF up to the moment of egg collection. After collection, the eggs are frozen. The aim behind freezing is to avoid the decline in egg quality that comes with ageing. In essence, it means that a woman can become her own egg donor later in life. However, if you are considering this, you need to understand that it isn't a fast fix or a guarantee.

Success rates reduce significantly with age. The highest live birth rates come from women who freeze eggs before they are thirty. In one recent study, the percentage of women who had a baby using their frozen eggs was 39 per cent of those who tried. These women had a median age of thirty-eight when they did egg-freezing. Those who froze their eggs under the age of thirty-eight had a success rate of 50 per cent. It's generally agreed that the best time to freeze eggs is under the age of thirty-six.

Women are advised, if possible, to freeze at least ten to fifteen eggs to give themselves a reasonable chance of a later pregnancy. This may often involve doing several rounds of treatment. However, even fifteen eggs may not be enough to give a good chance. Studies suggest that having at least twenty eggs to thaw can increase birth rates significantly. It's a good idea also to consider embryo-freezing using your partner's or donor sperm, as embryos have a much better freeze-and-thaw success rate, and doctors can tell much more about their quality than about that of an egg.

Egg-freezing does not offer any guarantees, but for a lot of women it presents a way to improve the chance of having their own biological children later in life. Women often report that it takes off the biological pressure to have a baby by a certain age and, by doing so, provides them with opportunities in life that they might otherwise not have had.

Surrogacy

Surrogacy involves a woman carrying and giving birth to a baby for another person or couple. The surrogate can act as the egg donor too, in what's referred to as 'partial surrogacy'. Any eggs and sperm have to undergo a screening process before they are used.

Surrogacy is used for women who don't have a womb, or whose womb makes it hard to carry a baby, or for women who are at risk of pregnancy complications. And it's used for single men, and men in couples. It's sometimes used when there have been multiple rounds of IVF without success or recurrent miscarriages.

The success rate of surrogacy depends on the quality of the eggs and sperm, the treatment (whether it's IUI/IVF/ICSI) and the health of the surrogate. In the UK a surrogate can either be a family member, a relative or a friend, or a volunteer found via an organization such as SurrogacyUK. Ideally, she will be under the age of forty and will have had her own children.

Surrogates cannot accept payment in the UK, aside from expenses related to being pregnant and loss of earnings. In some countries, surrogates are allowed to accept payment. It's important that all parties involved undergo counselling and that there's agreement on issues such as future contact, as well as a legal agreement in place.

Adoption

This is not ART, but it's included here because it can be a beautiful way to create a family. Choosing to adopt may be something people feel drawn to do, regardless of their fertility. Others come to adoption after unsuccessful rounds of IVF or pregnancy losses, or choose to adopt because they don't want to have ART. The adoption process involves in-depth screening and, if you've been undergoing fertility treatment, adoption agencies normally request that you abstain from trying for at least six months prior to applying to adopt.

TCP for ART

Optimize your general health and well-being with TCP, especially if you have coexisting medical conditions, for at least three months (ideally more) prior to starting ART, and continue throughout ART. You can also customize TCP by doing the following:

* **Ensure you have some sort of support system in place**, because ART can be emotionally draining. Many natural attempts at conception, followed by ART, will (even if you are resilient) be stressful. Address this regularly, communicating your feelings with your partner if you're in a couple, or with a friend or relative if you're single.

* **See a counsellor or therapist to help you to integrate more difficult emotions**. The holistic treatments and journaling in TCP can be helpful. There are also some great online and in-person communities where people share their experiences and support one another.

* **Read the advice in Chapter 12** if you have had unsuccessful IVF cycles or have experienced baby loss.

❋ **Keep an open mind**: the road to parenthood can be complex and filled with obstacles. I often see patients change their minds about a treatment or route they initially felt would not suit them.

❋ **Important as it is to know when it's appropriate to move on to ART, it's equally important to know when to re-evaluate or stop**: this can be very difficult when the emotions are strong. A counsellor can help, as can prioritizing your well-being. TCP can help you to gain clarity over this decision.

❋ **Be kind to yourself**: you're a human being doing the best you can with what you have, so show compassion to yourself and appreciation for all that you've done to get here.

CHAPTER 15

TCP for reproductive conditions

The final four chapters of the book cover how some reproductive conditions affect fertility, divided into conditions that affect the womb, the ovaries, the Fallopian tubes and the vulva, vagina and cervix. I'd encourage everyone to read these chapters, because looking after the environment of your reproductive organs is important for your overall health, but especially when it comes to conceiving, whenever that may be for you. These chapters are particularly relevant if you have the specific conditions listed under each chapter, though they are by no means limited to these alone:

* **Chapter 16, TCP for womb conditions**: endometriosis, adenomyosis, fibroids, uterine polyps, uterine malformations, menstrual-cycle disorders, heavy menstrual bleeding and chronic pelvic pain.

* **Chapter 17, TCP for ovarian conditions**: PCOS, ovarian cysts, irregular ovulation and oestrogen dominance (see page 110).

* **Chapter 18, TCP for Fallopian-tube conditions**: pelvic inflammatory disease, Fallopian-tube damage or scarring and ectopic pregnancy.

* **Chapter 19, TCP for conditions of the vulva, vagina and cervix**: vaginismus, vulvodynia, cervical disease such as cervical dysplasia (cellular abnormalities on the cervix).

In each of these chapters I'll suggest ways to add to your existing 12-week plan so that it's even more helpful to your specific case. Obviously medical management is important for all of these conditions – that goes without saying – but this book is about understanding that there is a lot you can do to help yourself, on top of medical advice and treatment.

The reason I've included four chapters on conditions that can affect reproduction is that trying to get pregnant when you have something such as endometriosis, PCOS or pelvic inflammatory disease can feel like a series of difficult barriers to overcome. Every time you have a symptom, such as pain or heavy bleeding, it reminds you that something isn't quite right. You may have been told that you need to get your body into a better and more receptive state, for pregnancy to happen naturally, or that you'll need to have fertility treatment. But very little advice is ever given on what you can do to help with this, let alone that the mind is a vital part of it. This is where TCP comes in. It views disease not just as a physical process, but as an emotional one too.

The medical treatment that's out there is often very limited. It's frustrating if you have a reproductive health condition, because historically there has been a lack of research into this area, meaning that treatments are often suboptimal and/or come with significant side-effects.

It's especially frustrating because the most common medical treatment for the last few decades has been to control a woman's menstrual cycle synthetically. This is most often done by prescribing one of the hormonal contraceptives. These not only prevent pregnancy – which is desperately unhelpful when you're trying to get pregnant – but have other downsides too (which I discuss on page 27), including a reduction in libido and a diminishment in sexual arousal. Although these treatments may relieve symptoms for a while, they do so while masking what's going on inside you. Whether hormonal contraception is being used to treat PCOS, endometriosis or heavy menstrual bleeding, it won't cure you. The underlying problem will persist. Indeed, it's common for women to discover they have a condition that may impact on their reproductive potential only after coming off the pill.

Hormonal contraceptives, though a useful treatment, sell women short unless they're specifically wanting to be on a contraceptive. I've found that most women, when offered the chance, want to engage with understanding their bodies better and what they can do in the long term to help themselves. When you have very difficult and upsetting symptoms, it's only natural that you want to find a way to stop them. But by teaching yourself to listen and understand their hidden messages, you have an amazing chance to learn about your body and how it works, to understand your cycle, get to know its rhythms and interpret its messages. And hopefully to discover the positive habits, such as good nutrition, exercise, sleep and stress management, that will help alleviate your symptoms and improve your natural fertility, without necessarily having to rely on external sources of hormones.

Another issue that I come across frequently is women feeling disempowered about their condition. The usual medical view is that these diseases are driven partly by genetics and, for the rest, by random events. As the causes are made to seem out of your control, treatment is too. In fact women are often told there's not much they can do to help themselves. Or that having a condition like PCOS or endometriosis will make it very difficult for them to become pregnant. When this becomes ingrained as a core belief, especially from a young age, this in itself may even contribute to infertility, as we have seen how powerfully emotions can affect cell behaviour.

This feeling of helplessness is compounded by the fact that, as females, we're expected to put up with such symptoms. Millions of women live with pain or heavy and unpredictable bleeding. We've been conditioned to believe this is a normal part of being a woman and that there's little that can be done to help. But these are patriarchal myths that have kept women enslaved by, rather than in charge of, their bodies. We need more funding into research that explores the connection between the mind and the body, as well as better education and awareness of what we can do to help ourselves.

I take a very different view of treating reproductive symptoms from the usual allopathic one, based on the premise of self-empowerment. Ideally, all girls and women would be educated earlier in life about how they can influence their fertility, their reproductive health and their well-being, as explained in TCP. But you can start now too: TCP tells you that you have the power to change; you can encourage your body to heal, with lifestyle modifications, but also by unearthing and processing your emotions and by dealing with any residual trauma you may have accumulated. It's all based on believing that your body is not broken and is always acting in your best interests. And that, given the right support, it can heal.

I see women having the most incredible innate instincts when it comes to their bodies. It's just that we end up ignoring these a lot of the time, because society teaches us to doubt our bodily wisdom. My advice, especially if you have a particular condition, is to keep checking in with your body and your instincts. Monitor your cycle as part of the 12-week plan; there is an additional exercise on this in Chapter 16. Do not ignore any symptoms, and do take notice when something doesn't feel quite right. Know that *you* are the best barometer of your own health. And never, ever feel bad about going to see a doctor and asking to be assessed.

Healing the microbiome to treat reproductive conditions

Hormones control so much of female health, but as you've learned, when they go wrong, it's a result of other, upstream imbalances that you have some control over, via the pillars of TCP. One of the keys is the body's microbiome. You know from Chapter 6 that what you eat can impact on your gut microbiome, and so also on your fertility.

When the microbiome is out of balance (called dysbiosis) it's been shown to contribute to the development of gynaecological conditions that affect reproduction, including PCOS and endometriosis. The make-up of the microbiome can impact on hormone levels, in particular oestrogen, but also progesterone, so much so that it's even been called an 'extended endocrine organ'. It's believed that the microbiome affects gene expression and therefore the absence or presence of disease, making it an important epi marker.

Let's take PCOS as an example. Like many reproductive issues, it involves a complex interaction of factors, making it very hard to unpick. But according to recent research, the microbiome seems to be key. It's thought that exposure to excess androgens (male hormones that women have too) in the womb can affect the foetal gut microbiome, among other things, predisposing a girl to developing PCOS later in life. Starting in the womb, the microbiome has an epigenetic influence on overall health and fertility. We know that in adult women, the overall diversity of the gut microflora is reduced in those who have PCOS, and this lack of diversity and dysbiosis contribute to inflammation, faulty blood-sugar control and associated obesity.

Good bacteria produce short-chain fatty acids (SCFAs), which support immunity and keep inflammation down, as well as controlling oestrogen levels. And the gut is where some key neurochemicals are made: peptide YY (a fullness hormone) and ghrelin (a hunger hormone), which are both lower in women with PCOS. Both of these mechanisms may contribute to the abnormal signalling that leads to the various hormonal, immune and neurological changes that we see with PCOS.

But the gut microbiome isn't the body's only microbiome. Although they tend to be smaller, there are populations of microorganisms living on the surface of your body and inside too. That includes in the vagina, but also the womb, the Fallopian tubes and the ovaries, making up around 9 per cent of your overall microbes. We can affect this microbiome too, even with simple things such as what we eat, what we wear and any contraceptives that we use.

You may know that vaginal infections, such as bacterial vaginosis (BV) and yeast infections, result from an imbalance in the vagina's delicate ecosystem. A balanced vaginal microbiome has been shown to have more of a bacteria called lactobacillus, which also protects against pelvic inflammatory disease (PID). Although yeast infections are often seen as innocuous, chronic untreated yeast overgrowth is associated with the release of toxins with far-reaching effects, impacting on hormonal balance, causing fatigue and contributing to infertility and autoimmune disease, as well as IBS.

The microbiome of the upper reproductive tract has been studied less, but it's known that it can be affected by bacteria that enter via the cervix, and by oral bacteria that can spread through intercourse. Several conditions have been linked with microbial imbalance in the upper reproductive tract, including endometriosis and PCOS (again), dysfunctional uterine bleeding, polyps (in the womb), PID, vulvodynia (persistent pain in the vulva) and cervical disease. Research has shown that where endometrial microbes were dominated by non-lactobacilli,

women undergoing IVF were less likely to have successful implantation, pregnancy and an ongoing pregnancy.

HOW TO NURTURE HEALTHY MICROBIOMES

* **Avoid:** synthetic and restrictive underwear, irritants
  in bubble baths, deodorants and perfumed, synthetic
  sanitary products, as well as repeated courses of
  antibiotics.
* **Eat an anti-inflammatory and vegetable-rich diet**
  (see page 80) and take steps to control stress (see
  Chapter 8).
* **Probiotics may help too:** in the gut they can increase
  the production of beneficial SCFAs and may also
  help to balance sex hormones in PCOS.

Trauma, emotions and reproductive conditions

As we've discussed, symptoms are really the body's only way of drawing our attention to unprocessed emotions or unhelpful thoughts and
beliefs, which we would otherwise continue to ignore. That's why we
can't separate the subject of menstruation and reproductive health
from that of managing our emotions and any associated stress. The
solution isn't simply to treat isolated symptoms or physical imbalances, but also to address reproductive health in its widest context, as
TCP does.

Our emotions provide us with valuable information, a guide to what
is going on energetically and biologically for us. But if we follow what
many of us have been taught, and brush our emotions to one side
or push them down, we miss out on the chance to have these essential opportunities to communicate with our body. If we keep ignoring
them, they find a way of getting our attention – which is by causing
symptoms. And we may miss the chance to intervene before a disease
becomes manifest. As Bessel van der Kolk writes in *The Body Keeps the*

Score, 'trauma robs you of the feeling that you are in charge of yourself'. When it comes to healing, being able to restore that control is really important. And you are ultimately in charge of your own health.

It may seem unusual to explain and treat reproductive conditions in terms of emotions. You'll see that for each organ – and sometimes for a particular condition – I'll describe the emotional patterns that I've seen, from my experience, in hundreds of patients in clinic. As discussed in Chapter 3, research has shown that certain conditions are linked with particular personality traits, which become adaptations and survival strategies in response to previous experiences. Each health condition can have a personality that manifests in the cells and tissues of an organ (or organs). And this is often the organ whose meridians are associated with the energetic epicentre of these emotions.

I've seen how different organs of the reproductive system tend to be the repository for a specific kind of trauma, and this trauma shapes the way the patient lives in the present. That is, there is a kind of personality and/or experience that goes with specific conditions relating to each organ, which may be contributing to the disease that is expressing there. It's useful to become aware of this and start to become curious about what your condition may be telling you about your emotional past and patterns, because recognizing this can be the start of your healing and your path to wellness and fertility.

FERTILE INTERACTIONS

The interaction between the immune, endocrine and neuro-psychological systems is a finely orchestrated symphony, one that's under the influence of a whole range of epigenetic factors. The immune system can affect your mental state, which in turn can have an effect on your hormones and neurology. Equally, your psychological state can impact on your immunity, neurology and hormones. These systems are constantly interacting and speaking with one another, so every time you address one of the pillars of TCP, you impact on multiple systems, not just one. Your physical biochemistry is linked with your genes, and so anything you do (including thoughts that generate emotions) speaks to your endocrine glands and your genes, influencing these interconnections. It's getting this symphony in tune that can lead you towards better health and fertility.

Charting your emotional cycle

If you have started charting your cycle for the 12-week plan, you may have noticed how your menstrual cycle is affected by the emotions you are feeling (or ignoring), the stress you are under, how well you're treating yourself, how well you're eating and sleeping or how you feel about yourself. Your cycle is an amazing portal to learning more about yourself and connecting with your body's natural wisdom. You may have noticed that premenstrually, for example, specific emotions come up, such as anger. These are not something you should ignore or hide, but are real and important messages from your body about deep-seated emotions that need to be expressed and that you can work through (see the journaling prompts in Chapter 16). Problems with the menstrual cycle – whether it's irregular, painful, heavy or prolonged periods – though sometimes attributable to underlying physical causes, almost always reveal where our emotional patterns and beliefs are out of sync. They can also reveal our shadow aspects, such as our difficulty in embracing emotions, discomfort over the attributes that make us female or our belief that sexuality or menstruation is shameful.

As the menstrual cycle is strongly affected by the endocrine glands and hormones, and as these are so closely intertwined with our energetic body and biofield, the different stages of a menstrual cycle also closely reflect our emotional patterns. In the first half of the cycle (the follicular phase) the focus is on building and growing, predominantly orchestrated by oestrogen, and many women report that this is the time when they feel energetic and have more stamina, as well as being more externally oriented in the world. If conception is to occur, it happens at ovulation, and the second half of the cycle following on from this (the luteal phase) is when women typically report feeling more emotionally labile, introspective and needing to spend more time on their own. This phase is ruled by progesterone, and emotions that may have been repressed can come up for processing, as they are encouraged to flow. Menstruation is a time when there's effectively a rebirth process, when new emotions can replace old ones and there's reintegration. You'll be doing an exercise in Chapter 16 that will help you reconnect with these different aspects of the menstrual cycle.

We discussed in Chapter 5 how trauma can become embedded in the body and can eventually manifest as infertility. It can also manifest as reproductive conditions. As an example, let's look at vulvodynia – a chronic, apparently unexplained burning or searing pain at the opening of the vagina. Around 10–25 per cent of women may experience this, and it's the leading cause of pain during sex (some women also experience it at other times, outside intercourse). The exact mechanism behind its development isn't clear. We know that it's physically associated with a history of infections, or with injured nerves and allergies.

However, vulvodynia is interesting because it's a physical condition of the reproductive organs that conventional medicine *does* accept has a psychological trigger or contributor. It's known that there's a strong association between abuse experienced during childhood and the onset of the condition. And there's a link to other kinds of early experiences associated with a lack of safety, such as neglect. Adverse experiences earlier and later in life are also important when it comes to many other conditions affecting reproduction: they all have an emotional underpinning, yet for the most part this isn't recognized by allopathic medicine. Because our reproductive organs have such a strong connection with our nervous and meridian systems, this is where trauma and unprocessed emotions tend to be stored and expressed.

The kind of trauma that very often comes up as the root of reproductive conditions is the Mother Wound, which you learned about in Chapter 5. The Mother Wound is the societal and familial control that comes from living in a patriarchal society, where shame and suppression are used to keep women feeling small. It's passed down the matrilineal line, from mother to mother (see Chapter 5 for more on this).

The Mother Wound propagates the fallacy that in order to succeed at life, you have to ignore your inner needs and desires. The core belief is that being a woman is difficult and leaves you vulnerable. I often see this presenting in a woman as a subtle ambivalence around mother-hood, where she wants a child, but isn't sure she will be a good parent; or is scared that her child will experience what she did, not feeling safe or supported in the world.

Looked at from a spiritual perspective, the reproductive organs are the birthing and creative centre of our body. They are bound up with both the root and sacral chakras, which are the source of who we are, how we show up in the world and how safe we feel there. Most women would agree that we have challenges in these areas, just by virtue of our common experiences of being gaslit, denigrated, abused, maltreated, outcast or denied a voice.

All women experience emotional trauma at some point in their lives, whether it's bullying, undermining, sexual assault, blame, judge-ment, discrimination or stigmatization. And so this part of us – our deep creative centre – is where we store the psychological scars of our personal experiences or those of the generations of women before us.

We have also absorbed the message that the female body is somehow imperfect, that menstrual blood is something to be hidden, that sexual-ity is either too much or not enough. Our conditioning and experiences not only lead to dysregulation of the stress response (see Chapters 5 and 8), but also to a biochemical environment that contributes to dys-regulation of our reproductive system and can, eventually, present as a condition. This is how the values passed down generationally – and all of our beliefs and traumas – end up having biological consequences on fertility, menstruation and ovulation.

More on healing the Mother Wound

A lot of the journaling prompts in the 12-week plan, and in this sec-tion, speak to healing the Mother Wound as well as your relationship with your mother. One of the first steps is learning to separate your own thoughts, beliefs and values from those of your mother. Beth-any Webster, author and transformational coach, describes how the responsibility you felt for your mother's pain may have stopped you from pursuing your own dreams, and that you may have done this because you wanted to be loved. Journaling will help you understand your own role, as well as your mother's role. It will help you grieve the relationship you may never have had with your mother, and to forgive yourself and her when you acted out of a sense of obligation rather than authenticity. During this process it's normal to grieve the pain that our mothers endured from their own Mother Wound. And to grieve the pain we may have suffered, as a result of being faithful to their pain. Once you feel the pain and understand its source, this allows its grip to lessen, which is the beginning of healing. And by doing this healing on a personal level, you may also initiate a healing within your mother too.

MEDITATION TO HELP TO HEAL THE MOTHER WOUND

Say the following meditation to yourself: 'I attune to the female maternal cell, the starting cell from my mother when she was a foetus herself. I clear from this cell all ancestral maternal genes and align this cell with Mother Earth. I thus encode into the cell lineage the ability to receive something in the future.

'I attune to the male paternal germ cell, which was the original germ cell in my father when he was a foetus. I clear all paternal ancestral genes from this cell to align it to the cosmos and incoming energies. I thus keep my present physical body aligned to new energies in the moment now.

'I visualize the male and female germ cells (sperm and egg cells) merging to fertilize myself as an embryo. I feel how much creativity and newness there is encoded in this union. I visualize that the whole of the spiritual world can sense the formation of the new Me.

'I ask to feel any unresolved, unfinished experiences and karma that would otherwise hold me back from my present purpose. I thus visualize all karma and unresolved business being completed, and align myself to new possibilities that I co-create with the Universe.'

That fibroids are linked with stress and trauma, for example, is shown by the way they disproportionately affect women of colour. As the author and psychotherapist Resmaa Menakem writes in *My Grandmother's Hands*, racism is rooted in our bodies and our nervous system. It is trauma caused by the cumulative effect of history, social systems and daily injustices. Patriarchal societies shame and oppress people and especially women. If you are a woman of colour, you'll likely have experienced this from birth, as well as being attacked and discriminated against for the colour of your skin, denied the same opportunities as someone who's white and/or having had to live in a state of hypervigilance to preserve your own safety or that of your family. Your ancestors will probably have been subjected to brutal forms of discrimination and violation. You will likely have experienced regular microaggressions as part of your daily existence, such as someone commenting on your skin or your hair, which can become traumatic when they accumulate.

There is also racism in how women of colour are treated within the medical system, in particular when it comes to reproductive conditions, birth and infertility. For example, a disproportionate number of women of colour do not have access to treatment for infertility. With this history of systemic trauma, is it any wonder that fibroids and Fallopian-tube diseases, as well as PCOS, are higher in women of colour?

Almost all women live with repressed emotions and culturally conditioned beliefs that can keep us stuck in abusive relationships or stop us from seeking opportunities, standing up for ourselves or calling out inappropriate or wrongful behaviour. But if we don't change this pattern, it will affect the next generation of women too. We can start by reclaiming and expressing our emotions and looking at our personal and collective trauma. On its own it's not a 'cure' for fertility problems. But it is the way we can deal with the most-upstream causes of women's overactive stress systems, which have a knock-on effect on all other systems too, including fertility. This is work worth doing, not just for ourselves, but for future generations too.

CHAPTER 16

TCP for womb conditions

The womb is the first and most important environment for a baby. As we have discussed, lifestyle choices epigenetically affect this environment and so they will shape a baby's future health, even beyond their genetic blueprint. And this influence carries over the generations; remember, when your mother was in your grandmother's womb, you were an egg cell inside your mother's ovaries.

For centuries, women's wombs have been used against them. Women have been labelled as 'hysterical' when they didn't comply with the patriarchal values of obedience and conformity. At a spiritual level, disease in the womb is often the misogyny of the world manifesting in our bodies. You could say that it's the Mother Wound expressed at a physical level.

In my work, two of the three most common conditions that I come across are to do with the womb: endometriosis and fibroids (the third is PCOS, see page 296). When looked at from a biological level, there isn't a single cause for most reproductive conditions, including endometriosis, but also other major womb conditions that affect fertility. Most womb conditions – fibroids, endometriosis, polyps – are responsive to hormones and are caused by multiple cellular changes as a result of epigenetic programming triggered by the local environment, affecting gene behaviour and leading to disease development. For example, we know that in endometriosis around 50 per cent of the condition is inherited – some of this will be genetic and some epigenetic. Yet, as we have so much control over our epigenome, it begins with a particular environment created in the body, which leads to epigenetic changes that drive the expression of the endometriosis genes, which in turn leads to the abnormal cell behaviour that results in the condition.

The epigenetic underpinning of womb conditions – including endometriosis and fibroids – explains why the holistic methods of

TCP pillars and the 12-week plan can help. They impact on epi mark-ers and so can positively impact on the course of the disease, even reducing or eliminating the need for medication.

Endometriosis

In endometriosis, tissue that is similar to the lining of the womb and has migrated around the body inflames and bleeds in response to hormonal, neurological and immune signalling. It's a multisystemic condition: the main symptoms are chronic pelvic and abdominal pain, but also heavy and painful periods, painful intercourse (dyspareunia), bladder and bowel symptoms, abnormalities to posture and the pelvic floor (due to adhesions), as well as chronic fatigue. Endometriosis can affect the gut, liver metabolism and bladder. And it alters gene expression in the brain that leads to remodelling and pain sensitization (see the box on page 280), along with mood disorders. Four out of five of women affected have mental-health issues – most commonly depression. Endometriosis has an association with autoimmune conditions, fibromyalgia and ME, all of which also have a strong mind–body connection. It's been estimated that a woman with symptomatic endometriosis may resort to using up to fourteen different medications to help control her symptoms.

Up to half of all women with endometriosis struggle to become pregnant. Pain can stop women from wanting or having sex. Endometriosis can damage Fallopian tubes, reduce the chances of fertilization and implantation and damage sperm. The inflammation associated with endometriosis can affect the ovarian reserve and accelerate the ageing of eggs. Having endometriosis can also increase the risk of pregnancy loss, and of pregnancy-related complications associated with the placenta, such as pre-eclampsia, low-lying placenta, small babies and preterm birth. All of these are linked with a maternal experience of trauma (see Chapter 5), and in fact research is beginning to discover a potential connection between maternal trauma and stress and the development of endometriosis in the child. It's possible that a significant number of cases that we currently refer to as 'unexplained infertility' could in part be due to endometriosis. A 2008 study by the Belgian gynaecologist Thomas D'Hooghe involved 221 laparoscopies on women who were infertile, but without any obvious symptoms. What he found was that close to 50 per cent had endometriosis, and 40 per cent of those had severe forms of the condition.

CASE STUDY

Roxie came to see me aged twenty-eight, when she and her partner had been trying to conceive for fourteen months. Her periods had always been painful and heavy, and she suffered from dyspareunia (pain during sex). After previous laparoscopy (keyhole surgery), she had been diagnosed with endometriosis as well as adenomyosis, where the endometrial cells that line the inside of the womb invade the muscle layer of this organ. These cells can swell, inflame and bleed, causing some of Roxie's symptoms. She also had a bicornuate uterus – an irregularly-shaped womb that occurs as a baby's organs are forming – and, though uncommon, this is slightly more common in women who have endometriosis and those who are affected by infertility.

Roxie was following most of the positive TCP habits: she knew how to look after herself, as she ate well, exercised and meditated regularly. But her emotional history revealed a difficult relationship with her mother, who was often absent and put pressure on Roxie to be an achiever. In combination with the difficulties she faced in her career as an aspiring actress, this contributed to her feeling that she wasn't ever good enough, which was compounded by unprocessed grief over an early miscarriage that she had experienced several years before.

Roxie was worried about having a bicornuate uterus, despite having been advised that it didn't require surgical intervention at this stage. I explained that, in spite of the slightly higher chance of miscarriage and preterm birth, along with a few other pregnancy-related complications, with close monitoring many women with this condition do go on to carry their babies to full term. We also talked about the emotional roots of uterine malformations and endometriosis. Women with uterine malformations often have a common underlying issue of unfinished business and residual anger towards people who have controlled or manipulated them in the past. Their goals and dreams have frequently been sacrificed for others. They may have felt manipulated into roles that they came to resent. It's as if they have had to twist and contort to fit someone else's idea of what they should be.

All of this was true of Roxie, who had sacrificed her own aspirations for the sake of her mother's love and approval, and it was a pattern also followed by Roxie's mother with her own mother. This intergenerational Mother Wounding had been passed on, potentially manifesting in Roxie's womb. I recommended a counsellor to explore all these issues, alongside rejection, abandonment and an eroded sense of self-esteem – other emotional themes that affected Roxie, and which are often associated with endometriosis.

As well as therapy, Roxie tried shamanism and kinesiology to help to engage her with old feelings that had been buried a long time ago, as a means of coping. She started seeing an osteopath too, to help relieve muscular and fascial tension around her organs; and an acupuncturist to help manage her stress and improve her period symptoms. She is continuing to invest in her well-being and fertility via the TCP pillars and is on the path towards wanting to conceive naturally.

‖‖

Endometriosis is driven by many of the mechanisms described in the first half of the book, a series of vicious cycles (see Chapter 5). There's an inflammation–hormonal cycle, where inflammation down-regulates genes that lower oestrogen production, which leads to higher oestrogen and subsequent endometrial tissue growth and proliferation, which in turn drives further inflammation. So the more inflammation you have, the more oestrogen you produce, and this can aggravate the symptoms of endometriosis.

There's also a stress–inflammation–pain cycle. Stress causes neurological and hormonal imbalances that create an environment of generalized inflammation (see Chapter 8) that leads to more stress and pain, plus a worsening of symptoms.

There's a trauma–epigenome cycle too. Like Roxie, women with endometriosis often have early traumatic experiences (see page 60). In particular, in common with women who have all kinds of womb conditions, the Mother Wound (see page 66) is key. There's also often fear around expressing emotions in the face of judgement or control, which leads to emotional repression and stress that ultimately affects the epigenome (see Chapter 5).

To add insult to injury, there is a social–emotional–stress cycle in endometriosis too, due to medical gaslighting and a lack of awareness of how the condition develops. On average, it takes around seven to eight years to get a diagnosis, and during this time women are often made to feel that the symptoms are all in their head.

This often leaves women who have endometriosis with a deep belief that life in their body isn't safe, either because no one believes them or because their symptoms prevent them being able to have normal relationships. This puts them at risk of depression, anxiety, agoraphobia, PTSD, substance abuse and addiction, plus sleep disorders, reduced concentration, overwhelming fatigue and damage to their memory, with almost 80 per cent being affected by at least some of these psychological symptoms. The repressed trauma and self-denial that accompany this often become clear when I discuss the diagnosis with my patients; their initial reaction can be tearful because it's often the first time they feel genuinely heard, seen and validated.

Fibroids

With fibroids, there are different genes and epigenetic processes underpinning the condition, but the principles are similar: epigenetic changes lead to abnormal signalling, which affects the behaviour of certain genes, leading to the condition. In this case, it's disordered collagen deposition leading to benign masses of connective tissue that affect the womb. And research shows that, for fibroid development, these abnormal patterns are contributed to through diet, stress and emotions, in particular through an increased sensitivity to oestrogen.

Most women (estimated to be around 70 per cent) may develop fibroids, but not all of them will have symptoms. Fibroids can cause heavy and prolonged menstrual bleeding because they have a rich vascular supply and can interfere with the uterus being able to contract. Pain related to fibroids is caused by pressure on surrounding organs and can also be due to degeneration, where a fibroid outgrows its blood supply. Fibroids that project outside the womb are more likely to cause symptoms, including pain, but also a frequent need to urinate, constipation and bloating.

Larger-sized fibroids that penetrate deeper into the muscle of the womb, and those that project into the uterine cavity, are more likely to cause problems with conception, implantation and miscarriage. Fibroids may disrupt the passage of sperm into the Fallopian tubes. It's thought that cross-talk between fibroids and endometrial cells interferes with the contractions of the womb, and this may stop implantation. And this may also be the case during IVF.

There's evidence that microRNA, which can affect the expression of various genes, is dysregulated in fibroids. As we saw in Chapter 15, women of colour are more likely to develop fibroids. One reason may be differences found in microRNA expression, possibly from being exposed to more trauma in societies with a white bias. Women of colour also tend to have larger tumours at diagnosis, an earlier age at diagnosis and more severe symptoms, leading to a greater need for intervention and a higher chance of infertility.

How TCP can heal womb conditions

What can make a big difference to womb conditions is dealing with your emotional landscape and previous trauma, changing old patterns of reacting and the narrative you've been made to believe about yourself. As the womb is a place where we store a lot of our old trauma and wounding, unresolved and unfinished emotional pain can build up here. And, as we saw above, it's not only our own personal trauma that can embed itself here, but also that of our mothers and grandmothers. Their fears and conditioned biological responses can be passed on to us, as trauma related to being a woman. This is why the impact of any unresolved family relationship issues can often make their mark in the womb.

As the uterus lies in the centre of the pelvis it's related energetically to the second or sacral chakra. This is associated with the relationship you have with yourself, as well as the one you have with others in the world. And so relationship conflict and out-of-balance power dynamics, such as societal or familial manipulation, control, violation, suppression or shaming, can, over time, lead to dysfunction here. And this might manifest as difficult symptoms, for example pain and/or heavy bleeding, or even fibroids or endometriosis. It works best to look at these conditions holistically, treating and reducing stress, while correcting underlying energetic patterns, conflicts and emotional issues.

The behaviour of the cells and tissues often reflects what's happening in a woman's life and her emotional state. For example, take fibroids. The way they're seen bursting out of the usual confines of the wall of the womb symbolizes a need to break free from limitations. Many women with fibroids tend to reveal a history of being unable to fully express themselves in their lives, careers or relationship, and a need to cut loose from the limits imposed on them. And they may have had to suppress past anger, rage, sadness, grief, resentment and humiliation, for fear that expressing their emotions will have consequences.

The story of trauma underlying abnormal bleeding and polyps

If you have one of the womb conditions that involves excessive (see page 159) or painful bleeding, including fibroids and endometriosis, but also uterine polyps (see below), it's worth going deeper into underlying trauma. Abnormal bleeding may signal that there are traumatic emotions needing to be expressed. Tissue that haemorrhages is literally bleeding for our attention.

Abnormal bleeding is the most common symptom of uterine polyps (when they have symptoms). These are growths in the inner wall of the uterus. When it comes to fertility, polyps can sometimes interfere with implantation, depending on size and location, either mechanically or because they're associated with inflammation that creates a hostile environment. When polyps block the cervical canal or the entrance to the Fallopian tubes, they may block the passage of sperm too. And polyps can raise levels of inflammatory biochemical messengers, such as matrix metalloproteinase (MMP), which can be toxic to sperm and interfere with fertilization and implantation.

Women affected by uterine polyps have a similar behavioural profile to women with fibroids: they present strong protective defences to the world, while underneath they're dealing with loss, grief and trauma. Problems with implantation may be a biological reflection of these defences: a protection against someone or something getting too close. These women may fear that if they allow themselves to express the emotions they've been hiding, they will be abandoned or judged, and this may be due to people letting them down in the past.

As we've seen from all the typical emotional patterns related to womb conditions, the womb can either be a source of empowerment or disempowerment. This depends on how well we recognize and heal the Mother Wound and other trauma we may have been exposed to. The womb is highly responsive to the environment, moulding and adapting to changing circumstances that we create. And so if we can heal it, the womb has a great capacity for renewal, with its cells shedding and regenerating each month. It's a source of immense, creative, life-giving power and a potent source of connection to our maternal lineage (this is true energetically even for women who don't have a womb). Spiritually, it brings us the hope of rebirth and the potential of transformation. And TCP supports this capacity for regeneration.

DEALING WITH GYNAECOLOGICAL PAIN

In the past, women have often been gaslit about pain from endometriosis and other types of gynaecological pain. They have either been told it can't be as bad as they think it is, they don't need treatment and/or they need to learn to live with it. Many women therefore live on painkillers, some of which can not only be addictive, but have significant side-effects.

Pain management works best when considered holistically, especially given what we now understand about how pain works. For example, endometriosis pain is amplified via new neural connections and brain remodelling, causing sensitization of pain pathways alongside persistent activation of the stress response. The pain signals from nerve endings feed into the limbic system in the brain, where we process emotions and memories; the brainstem, which is responsible for our stress response; and the cerebral cortex, which oversees all inputs to the brain. This effect on the brain is like the volume on the pain-dial being turned up. It leads to emotional distress, mental-health issues and a greater sensitivity to pain, as well as more intense memories of pain.

You may find it helpful to change the narrative around your pain. Ask yourself: what is the pain trying to show me and tell me? Close your eyes and say out loud the words you normally use to refer to your pain or your body. Notice whether they activate fear or other feelings. Where in the body do you feel those emotions? Are there particular images associated with them?

What more positive and compassionate terms could you use to replace these words? For example, consider replacing the word 'pain' with 'waves', or 'it hurts' with 'it's leading me towards greater awareness and self-compassion'. Try saying these out loud. Notice the difference in how this makes you feel.

Journaling for womb conditions

Ideally, you should do this every day of your cycle, or at least for each of the different phases: follicular, ovulation, luteal and menstrual. It's a beautiful way to reflect and integrate the wisdom of each phase. The idea is to look back over the weeks and then months to find the patterns that occur at different stages of your cycle, and then to reflect on what they may be telling you. As you do TCP and continue to journal, you can think about what has changed and is changing, and how.

Menstruation is a particularly powerful time. Traditionally thought to occur in sync with the new moon (though women can menstruate at different phases of the moon), it's a time when women go through a period of darkness to face their shadows and restore, regenerate and renew. In native cultures, menstruation was seen as spiritual. Those who are menstruating become much more receptive, as well as sensitive to things we wouldn't normally notice.

Periods have been 'taboo' for many generations, whereas originally the meaning of this word and periods themselves were sacred, although in our patriarchal societies both have become distorted and associated with shame. We need to be aware of this and the emotional pain and shame that we've internalized around the menstrual cycle, so that we can change the narrative we pass on to our children and future generations.

Menstruation can be deeply emotional. Many women may find themselves, especially in the lead-up to their periods, with changeable moods, suddenly feeling overwhelmed with sadness or rage. Hormones do affect mood directly, but another reason is that some of the memory and emotional parts of the brain remodel during menstruation, and there are changes in the interaction between the two brain hemispheres. Again, many of us have been made to feel ashamed of these feelings and to hide them, even from ourselves. But they provide subconscious clues as to where in our lives we need change to occur. Uncomfortable or painful issues that arise now need to be listened to, and it's important to express them, even if only in a journal as a beginning.

At this potent time, when you have far greater access to your intuition than at any other moment, it's natural to withdraw and spend time with yourself. You may need this to deal with the emotions that come up, even without menstrual cramps or heavy bleeding. By attuning to your body and honouring your cyclical needs, you can become better at setting boundaries and getting the rest you need, so that you're the best version of yourself, rather than depleted and exhausted. This will also help you develop gratitude for the powerful messages that your body is capable of communicating, given enough time and space.

Instead of being shamed and ridiculed over emotions that arise during the menstrual cycle, women and girls need to start being honoured and heard.

Day of cycle (Day 1 is first day of bleeding)

Write down in your journal your responses to the following prompts:

* **Moon time**: the phase the moon is in, whether full, new, waxing or waning.

* **Nutrition**: what are the foods you're craving now? How do you feel after eating those foods? Are there any that you find help your symptoms or your mood?

* **Exercise**: what exercises are you most drawn to now? Do they leave you feeling energized or depleted? Do you feel able to take on the challenges of exercise or do you feel you need to be gentler with yourself, to do something less strenuous?

* **Stress**: is there any particular stress affecting you now? How is it making you feel, and what impact is it having on you? How are you sleeping? Can you recall any dream you may have had and what it was about? Was it a recurring dream? Are there any particular thoughts that you're ruminating over?

* **Physical changes**: have you noticed any changes such as breast tenderness, tummy swelling or bloating, an alteration in your bowel habit or a change in your libido? Any other symptoms or experiences?

* **Sexuality and relationships**: how have you found yourself communicating with people in your life (your partner/family/ friends)? Have any particular issues been affecting you? Are you feeling sociable, or do you crave being alone? How aligned is your work at this time to your needs? Are you able to express your needs to your colleagues, friends and

family or partner? What is your relationship with yourself like? Are you craving sex and touch or is there resistance to engaging with this?

MENSTRUAL-CYCLE MEDITATION

Say the following meditation to yourself: 'I attune to the vibrations during the menstrual cycle.

'Thus I attune to the vibration of the first two weeks of the cycle, while the uterus lining is building up. I visualize that this is the phase when my body is laying into the uterus energies that provide the future nest of the baby. I sense to what extent my personal history and my physical body's memories are incorporated into the uterine lining. I visualize clearing all personal blueprints from the uterus, to free the energy and allow the uterus to hold the appropriate nurturing energy for the embryo without any of my distortions. I attune to the vibration of oestrogen released from my ovaries during this time and sense this is responsible for the building-up forces at this time.

'I then visualize that the history of the world, and all physical life and evolution that has ever existed on Earth, is encoded in my ovaries, egg cell and is laid into the uterus lining. I sense this creates a proper nest for the embryo. I then visualize that the moon's energy assists me in clearing all past vibrations from my uterus. I thus sense I am allowing my building-up energy in the uterus to be responsive to the spiritual and Earth energies entering into the present moment of conception.

'I attune to the vibration of ovulation when I sense there is an opening of a column of light through my spine and head centres into my reproductive system. I sense this influx of spiritual fire is the reason for the rise of my basal temperature at the time of ovulation.

'I attune to the vibration of the third week of my menstrual cycle, and visualize that this imparts a connection to the emotional life of the new incoming embryo soul. I attune to the vibration of the hormone progesterone, which is released from my ovaries and is active during this time, and sense it allows a connection between my energetic and my physical body. I visualize connecting to the embryonic soul.

'I sense to what extent I'm stuck in emotional patterns within myself, and clear these to allow for the incarnation process of a new baby.

'I then attune to the shedding of the menstrual blood in my period. I sense how easy or difficult it is to let go of the menstrual blood. I let go of what no longer serves me and allow reintegration to happen.

'I then attune to the vibration I have after my period, and sense how free and further aligned to Spirit I am.'

TCP advice for womb conditions

In addition to general TCP advice, here are some areas to focus on for womb conditions:

Nutrition

* **Eat most of your fruit and veg raw** to increase glutathione levels during ovulation and support egg development.

* **Eat sweet potatoes and leafy greens in the luteal phase of the cycle** to help to balance oestrogen and progesterone, and to counteract oestrogen dominance, supporting the liver in eliminating waste hormones.

* **Eat progesterone-rich foods**, such as salmon, cruciferous vegetables and nuts. Brown spotting before a period may be indicative of low progesterone levels.

✳ **Reduce egg-yolk consumption**, as these are rich in arachidonic acid and can increase inflammation and menstrual cramps if you suffer from these; opt for a white-egg omelette instead.

✳ **Eliminate trans fats**, as they increase inflammation and insert themselves into cell membranes, which can cause cell dysfunction and interfere with cell-signalling.

✳ **Eat more vegetables, lean protein, beans and nuts during the follicular phase**, when hormone levels are at their lowest; even consuming some oestrogen-rich foods such as soya is best done at this time.

✳ **Eat more fibre-rich foods, such as spelt and quinoa, during ovulation**, when oestrogen reaches a peak. Incorporate lots of vegetables and fruit for their antioxidant benefits, and lots of fibre to ensure that excess oestrogen is being appropriately metabolized.

✳ **Increase your natural progesterone levels during the luteal phase**, by consuming foods that promote progesterone production, such as cabbage, kale, broccoli, Brussels sprouts, spinach, wholegrains, pumpkin seeds, nuts, bananas and shellfish. This will also help to counteract any dominant oestrogen. Complex carbs, such as wholegrain bread, pasta and brown rice, are important at this time too, to help reduce mood swings.

✳ **Ensure that you eat more iron-rich foods during menstruation**, such as beetroot and organic meat as well as seaweed and seafood. Rather than eating food that is raw, this is the time to focus on cooking and eating stews and soups, as well as baked vegetables.

✳ **Eat avocados regularly**, as they contain indole-3-carbinol, which helps to bind excess oestrogen; as well as cruciferous vegetables such as cabbage, broccoli and Brussels sprouts that contain diindolylmethane, which also helps to modulate oestrogen levels.

❋ **Increase the fibre content of what you eat**, such as wholegrains, chia seeds, beans, brown rice and, of course, vegetables and fruit, which helps to eliminate excess hormones.

❋ **Some supplements may be helpful**: vitamins B, D and E have been shown to reduce PMS-related symptoms. Vitamin B also helps with natural progesterone production. Manage anaemia, if you suffer from heavy periods, by increasing your intake of iron-rich foods and, if needed, by supplementing with iron. Regular vitamin C has been shown to help reduce the amount of blood loss during menstruation. And vitamin E helps to reduce excessive clotting. Taking magnesium helps to relax smooth-muscle tissue and so is useful for easing uterine cramps. Herbal supplements can also be helpful to manage some conditions. However, if you are on medication or looking to conceive, speak to your doctor about these.

Exercise

❋ **Spend time in natural daylight and nature** to help regulate your hypothalamus, which relies on natural day- and night-rhythms to release various hormones and neurotransmitters.

❋ **Listen to what your body needs** and adjust your exercise according to the phases of the menstrual cycle (see Weeks 4 and 5 of the 12-week plan).

Stress

❋ **If you have a condition that affects your womb**, the pelvic-floor muscles and ligaments that hold up your uterus can end up pulling, pushing or creating tension that leads to misalignment. This can also change the position of various pelvic organs. Osteopathy and chiropractic adjustments can help with tension and blockages. Deep-tissue massage can help realign pelvic organs, release tension and stress and create space in the fascia (that wraps all the tissues in our body), to help restore blood and lymph flow, as well as nerve function. Acupuncture at ovulation and menstruation can help to restore meridian flow and hormonal balance. Reflexology and reiki can help to relieve PMS symptoms, pain and endometriosis symptoms.

* **Heat pads, warm baths and saunas** can help to promote circulation and relieve muscular tension and inflammation (this isn't recommended if you're actively trying to conceive or are pregnant).

* **Be disciplined about going to bed and getting up at the same time each day**, to help support the circadian rhythm that many hormones are dependent on.

* **Affirm to yourself that although chronic pain is an important message from your body**, it can also be seen as an opinion made by your body and, in itself, may not be dangerous. You can use visualization to reduce the perception and intensity of pain. Realize that chronic physical pain almost always has a wider context of stress or unprocessed emotions from past trauma. Know that emotions are safe in themselves. In time, journaling will help you move towards acceptance, understanding and safety.

* **Flare-ups of pain are natural when you have a hypervigilant dysregulated nervous system**, even during recovery, as the brain is forming new neural connections. Until these completely replace the well-established paths, old messages about pain will keep being reactivated.

* **Reduce your exposure to electromagnetic radiation –** which can lead to geopathic stress in the body and affect

the meridian system, which is closely linked with the endocrine glands – by having downtime from your phone and limiting Wi-Fi exposure in the house.

❊ **Treat constipation through diet and exercise** if you suffer from this, as it can interfere with eliminating excess hormones.

Relationships

❊ **Be accepting of, and kind to, yourself**: healing takes patience and regular perseverance. Encourage your body to heal by making positive assumptions and creating new belief patterns, such as 'My body can, and will, heal. I can pace myself each day. My body is not broken – it is always acting in my best interests.'

❊ **Nurture and send love to your inner child**, the part of you that longs to be safe, to connect, to be held, heard and seen, and to be loved. She is the child within you who may never have received the love she craved from her parents.

Habits to help heal the Mother Wound

❊ **Create a new relationship with yourself**, free from any expectations imposed on you by others.

❊ **Learn to mother yourself**, which is the act of meeting your adult emotional and physical needs.

❊ **Find the places in you that feel hurt or stuck** and give yourself the love that you didn't receive.

❊ **Build the capacity to meet all of your feelings without shame.**

❊ **Nurture the neglected and abandoned parts of you.**

❊ **Practise compassion for yourself.**

* **Heal your relationship with your mother** by holding a space for her and showing compassion for the difficulties she faced.

* **Recognize that your mother's emotional absence was not your fault**: if your mother wasn't there for you emotionally or was overly critical of you and your choices in life, understand that this wasn't because you weren't good enough or unlovable, or due to something you did.

* **Instead of seeing your mother as the person you want her to be**, see her as she is. When you accept that your mother was conditioned by her own inheritance and the cultural expectations that confined her as a woman, you can begin to accept her – even at times when she may not have been the mother you needed her to be – and true healing in your relationship with her can begin.

* **Practise loving-kindness towards yourself**: most of us are our own worst critics, and often the criticism stems from messages we've internalized from our parents or the world around us. When you notice criticism of yourself creeping in, stop and pay attention to where it seems to be coming from. Whose voice is it, and would you speak to your best friend or your child with those words and in that tone? Each time you stop and reflect, it'll become easier to autocorrect and, instead of criticizing, you'll find words of comfort and compassion for yourself.

OESTROGEN DOMINANCE (OD)

Oestrogen is a feel-good hormone, essential for fertility and well-being. But you can have too much compared to its counter-hormone, progesterone. Modern lifestyles tend to lead to the amplification of oestrogen and its effects all over the body. Some of the symptoms include cyclical breast tenderness, breast cysts, shorter menstrual cycles, earlier age of first period, heavy or irregular menstrual bleeding, PMS, menstrual migraines, and a predisposition to fibroids and endometriosis. It can even increase the risk of hormone-related cancers, such as breast cancer, and the chance of diabetes.

Oestrogen dominance doesn't tend to exist on its own, and neither does progesterone deficiency. They are both often a response to upstream imbalances that we have some control over. Cortisol, the main stress hormone, for example, is the principal upstream hormone that, when dysregulated, can lead to downstream hormonal side-effects, including oestrogen dominance. Another contributor is being overweight, because adipose tissue itself makes oestrogen. Oestrogen dominance may also be due to an imbalanced gut microbiome, poor liver function, a low-fibre and nutritionally imbalanced diet, disturbed sleep patterns and oestrogen-mimicking chemicals from the environment that can start to accumulate even before birth, due to the mother's exposure. The good news is that our bodies are incredibly resilient and you can undo, and even reverse, years of potential harm through changing lifestyle measures.

Many of the pillars of TCP will help to rebalance oestrogen and progesterone. Plenty of vegetables and fibre help support the microbiome, which is key in oestrogen metabolism, and also help eliminate excess oestrogen via the gut. Keep your bowel habit regular and avoid toxins (including plastic) to reduce the chemical load on your body. Managing stress via the techniques described in Chapter 8 is important, due to the impact of stress on the HPG axis (see page 108). You may also want to increase your intake of zinc, which helps to support natural detoxification pathways in the liver.

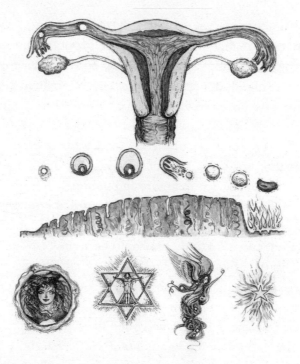

Esoteric physiology of the menstrual cycle by Katherine Mynott

The upper part of the image shows the overall layout of the female reproductive system. Two stages of an ovulated ovum are shown on the lefthand side, and stages of sperm transit shown from the high vaginal cavity towards the ovum as mid-fallopian tube level. The next row of images depicts stages of follicle development within the ovary and ovulation, followed by corpus luteum changes within the residual follicle at the ovary. The next lower image sequence shows the build-up of endometrial lining within the uterus, followed by stabilization or plateau stage and then menstrual shedding as the period in the fourth week. The lowest level of images shows spiritual aspects of the cycle. Earth Mother elemental energies on the left stream into the endometrial build-up and follicle development. The Star of David image symbolizes the ovulation mid-point as the opportunity for an incarnating soul to prepare to potentially connect to the germ cells. The maturation plateau phase of the cycle coincides with the angel figure, to represent the movement of the astral body through the sacral. Finally, the star with its heat radiations represents the ego becoming more active during the menstrual period itself.

CHAPTER 17

TCP for ovarian conditions

If you could hold a normal ovary, it would fit into the palm of your hand. And you'd see how it's dotted with follicles, little pouches that house the eggs and are filled with fluid that nourishes them.

You'd also see that an ovary looks a lot like a miniature version of a brain. And together with its twin, it acts a bit like one too: the ovaries are the main producers of sex hormones, which control a multitude of biological mechanisms and communications overseeing fertility and well-being. They're also directly connected to the brain. This means that, as an organ, they're a source of essential communication as well as life.

We're born with millions of eggs existing in a state of suspended animation, called meiosis. But even before we're born, egg numbers start to decline (see the ovarian reserve on page 240). Only a relatively small number are chosen to mature from immature primordial follicles to become dominant follicles and undergo ovulation. This process of folliculogenesis is highly selective. Those eggs that are recruited grow surrounded by follicular fluid, an ever-changing hormone soup overseen by the central nervous system, and the HPG axis (see page 31).

At any given point, the ovary contains follicles of a wide range of maturity level and sizes. Ideally, lifestyle change to prepare for conception should start a year beforehand, as this is when the follicle that may give rise to your future baby will begin folliculogenesis. But the most critical time consists of the three months before ovulation – the time between a follicle being recruited from storage and ovulation. This is the reason for TCP's 12-week plan.

The process controlling folliculogenesis and all its contributing factors is still to be discovered, but we do know that it's negatively affected by stress. The selection, and the integrity of the resulting eggs, is believed to be driven epigenetically. In other words, we may be able to optimize this through what we do via our lifestyle. And during that key three-month period the egg is under the influence of multiple epigenetic effects via its cell membrane, which is bathed in follicular fluid and fed by the blood supply of the ovary. The DNA of the egg won't change in response to its environment, but how it's read and expressed will. In addition to this, as different forms of stress have been shown to lead to dysfunction and a shortening of telomeres (the caps of DNA that keep it stable), we may possibly also be able to have an impact on the rate of ovarian ageing and even the onset of menopause through the way we live our lives.

The energetics of the ovaries

The ovaries have a dynamic energy. For the first two weeks of the cycle the dominant follicle grows. Then, when the egg bursts out of the follicle at fertilization, the follicle becomes the corpus luteum or yellow body and starts producing progesterone. If fertilization doesn't happen, the corpus luteum is absorbed by the ovary, along with the follicles that weren't chosen for ovulation. And so the ovaries are constantly changing throughout the cycle, growing follicles and re-absorbing them too.

The spiritual view recognizes ovaries as the source of our creativity. After all, the growth and release of an egg is the ultimate creation, giving rise to another human being. It depicts ovaries as the source of all creative manifestation, including writing, art and music as well as science, and as our barometer of how well the life force of creation flows and expresses in our lives.

Much like testicles for men, ovaries are the place where women are said to store their gumption and courage. They produce not only oestrogen and progesterone, but testosterone too, and so express both our masculine and feminine aspects. Ovarian problems can arise when the balance between male and female energies is disrupted by life, and we either become too assertive and aggressive in the pursuit of what we want or fall into states of victimhood.

CASE STUDY

A sense of victimhood was the case for Connie. When she came to see me, she and her partner had been trying to get pregnant for three years. Like a lot of women with PCOS, Connie was ovulating rarely. We talked about her symptoms and her irregular cycle. Then I asked about her upbringing. Connie told me that her mother was controlling, bossy and overbearing, always telling her what she should think and do. Since childhood, Connie had got into a pattern of playing small – the obedient and conforming daughter – in order to avoid conflict.

The pain of suppressing herself, of not being accepted for herself and of being unable to fully express her frustration and anger at being controlled had found an outlet in her body, expressing itself as PCOS. PCOS ovaries are described as having the appearance of a 'string of pearls'; they are enlarged by lots of immature follicles that have stopped growing at 5–8mm. And so her PCOS was manifesting her silent anger as these multiple small follicles waiting to burst, but never quite reaching the point of maturity. As we've already seen for womb conditions, the physical manifestation of a condition often has synergy with the emotional issues underlying it. Frequently the immature follicles of PCOS can also reflect an unexpressed creative part of the woman. Connie's physical symptoms were reflecting the limitations and control that her mother imposed upon her. At the same time, her body stopped ovulating and menstruating, regressing to when she was a little girl, which is exactly how she felt around her mother.

Once Connie committed to therapy, including counselling, shamanism and reiki, and learned ways to be more honest with herself and with her mother, her ovulation resumed. This wasn't the only factor in her recovery – as we'll see below, the other pillars are important in PCOS too – but it was an important part of restoring her health and wellness.

Inside PCOS

Up to one in five women may have PCOS (polycystic ovary syndrome). It's one of the top causes of infertility and the number-one cause of infertility related to irregular or absent ovulation (anovulation). Like other gynaecological conditions, including endometriosis (see Chapter 16), PCOS is multi-systemic: a neuroendocrine and metabolic condition involving the dysregulation of several organ systems that features abnormal signalling between the brain and the endocrine system, along with inflammation.

It's important to note that while a scan might reveal you have polycystic ovaries, this doesn't mean you'll have polycystic ovary *syndrome*. The syndrome often starts at puberty and, as well as polycystic ovaries, symptoms include blood-sugar dysregulation that can develop into diabetes, high blood pressure, excessive hair growth or hirsutism, irregular periods, problems with weight management and infertility. PCOS can cause problems with ovulation and implantation, and in pregnancy it can increase the risk of miscarriage, gestational diabetes and pre-eclampsia. But as women with PCOS have a higher overall anti-Müllerian hormone (AMH), pregnancies over forty are more common and the age of menopause is also thought to occur later. Women with PCOS are more at risk of other chronic health issues, such as endometrial cancer and problems with lipid metabolism leading to heart and vascular disease.

Hormonal issues include an imbalance between luteinizing hormone (LH) and follicle-stimulating hormone (FSH), problems with insulin sensitivity, plus higher androgen and AMH levels. All these factors may collude to mean that a dominant follicle might not develop and so ovulation doesn't happen or happens irregularly.

PCOS is a chicken-and-egg situation: it has a range of contributory factors, and its effects also drive the condition. Androgens make tissues more insulin-resistant. This upsets blood-sugar regulation, leading to inflammation. And inflammation produces more androgens by increasing cortisol, driving further insulin resistance as well as hormonal imbalances that affect the brain and interfere with how it signals with the ovaries, starting the whole cycle over again.

The psychological-stress aspects of PCOS probably feed into this too. Psychological stress isn't simply the consequence of the disease. It could be a significant contributing factor to it, via the HPG axis that you met in Chapter 2, the brain–reproductive connection. There are mental-health elements to PCOS: patients are five times likelier to suffer from anxiety, three times likelier to have depression, and more than 60 per cent of women with the condition have at least one psychological disorder, including obsessive compulsive disorder, bipolar disease and eating disorders.

It's thought that psychological distress may contribute to PCOS, and possibly also episodes of overeating and extreme dieting during puberty and adolescence. Mental and physical stress can oversensitize the HPG axis – the communication between the brain and the reproductive organs – and this may cause epigenetic changes to DNA that lead to PCOS.

A genetic tendency for PCOS seems to be inherited via the maternal lineage. Up to 70 per cent of girls born to women with PCOS will go on to develop the condition. Interestingly, sons can inherit a version of PCOS too, developing symptoms that reflect metabolic dysregulation, including diabetes, obesity and male-pattern baldness.

Mitochondrial-DNA abnormalities are also being investigated as possible causes of PCOS. Given what we understand about the association between the Mother Wound and mitochondria (see Chapter 5), it's possible that unresolved emotional issues stemming from the relationship with our mothers – and those before them – could be another contributor to the development of PCOS. We also know that mitochondria are the main power centres in cells, and looking after these through nutrition and exercise (see Chapters 6 and 7) is important, especially in a condition like PCOS.

Exposure to high levels of AMH as a foetus seems to cause the epigenetic changes that trigger PCOS later in life. Research shows that excess AMH injected into pregnant mice leads to their offspring developing features of PCOS, including infertility. There are other genes involved that, when epigenetically triggered, lead to symptoms. These include genes relating to neural growth, cell proliferation, inflammation and insulin signalling. Being exposed to elevated levels of androgens in the mother's womb can also make the HPG axis more sensitive to stress later in life, leading to dysregulated signalling between the brain and the ovaries.

Stress and inflammation can increase the production of androgens, and then high androgen levels can lead to obesity, insulin resistance and altered fat metabolism. This makes it hard to lose weight. Weight gain leads to a vicious cycle of high androgens, insulin resistance and further inflammation. However, there is a subtype of PCOS where weight gain isn't a feature. These are the one-third to half of women with PCOS who either have a normal or lower BMI. If this is you, the same TCP advice will still apply, but there is some variation with exercise that is described at the end of the chapter.

The emotional underpinning of ovarian issues

As the ovaries are related to the second energetic centre (sacral chakra), they have an intimate association with our relationships, both with others and with ourselves. This includes the one with our mother, which again makes the Mother Wound key, but also the relationships with our father, siblings, partner, friends and bosses. The ovaries' energies can become distorted when a woman isn't able to express the fullness of herself, whether due to constant criticism, being told she's not capable, being made to feel and act small, when she's undervalued and unappreciated for her contributions or manipulated and abused by those around her. And so exploitation, power struggles or denigration in any relationship have the potential to lead to ovarian disease.

The negative pattern may have begun as a dysfunctional relationship with parents that set up a longing for parental approval and pushed the woman towards seeking external validation. Ovarian problems are to do with constantly feeling the need to prove oneself or push oneself to an extreme to feel accepted, loved, desired or appreciated. In fact it's no wonder so many women suffer from ovarian disorders when the expectations set upon us are so impossible to reach. Society constantly puts pressure on women. Not only are we expected to be smart and pretty, but also polite, well presented, calm, perfect mothers and colleagues, as well as cleaners, chefs and all-round emotional and family counsellors.

As Connie's story shows, energetically there's often a sense of the woman feeling the need to conform or having to become strong or dependable from a young age, or having to become tough in order to survive. And women can end up adopting an excess of masculine qualities to do this. An ovary that is polycystic is bigger than usual with a hard and tough cortex, reflecting what is often happening at the emotional level. Ovarian disease tends to be associated with a leaning towards overdrive, overexertion, overachievement and over-compensation. Women who operate in male-dominated institutions are more prone to developing these traits, and given that most insti-tutions uphold patriarchal values, that means a lot of women are affected. They also tend to have people who are abusive and domi-neering in their life or in a relationship, such as a friend, colleague or relative. They have a fear of being shamed or judged. And they can have poor personal boundaries, due to overwhelm and unexpressed anger at being unable to stand up to the perpetrators. Their personal needs often conflict with the demands set upon them by the outer world. They can feel trapped between their natural desires and what they feel obliged to do.

PCOS has some additional emotional issues associated with it. If during puberty a girl has negative feelings about becoming a woman, because of beliefs that she may have internalized from her parents or from observing how other women are treated in the world, then the irregularity or absence of periods in PCOS may be a subconscious attempt to prevent this transition – really a denial of her womanhood.

Her feelings may have come from ambivalence around expressing her femininity, perhaps from seeing her mother maltreated, or from a perpetuated belief that women are the less capable sex, maybe as a result of suffering abuse herself or feeling vulnerable due to unwanted sexual attention or advances. She may have developed deep-seated fears and trauma about becoming a mother, and there may be ances-tral trauma inherited via a lineage of women who felt enslaved by their role in life. The result of this pattern is often anger, frustration and resentment that lodges in the ovaries.

Women with PCOS frequently have a complicated relationship with their sexuality, either because of previous abuse or violation or from seeing other women suffer this. They may build a wall of defences in order to feel safe. Previous abandonment issues may have also led to defensiveness and reluctance to allow others to get too close, for fear they may be taken advantage of or let down. As mentioned previously, polycystic ovaries are typically stiffer, larger and harder, reflecting the fact that the woman has often had to become tougher in order to survive in a male-dominated world.

Understanding ovarian cysts

CASE STUDY

I met Gabby when she was thirty-five, when she came to see me about a cyst on her ovary. There are various kinds of cysts; the kind that Gabby had isn't the same as those of PCOS. Gabby's was 6cm in size on her right ovary and was called a 'dermoid cyst', the most common non-cancerous ovarian cyst in women under the age of forty, which can contain a variety of different tissues as a result of forming from cells initially destined to develop as eggs or sperm. Her cyst was causing abdominal bloating and increasingly frequent bouts of pelvic pain, especially during sex.

Some ovarian cysts are normal and go away in one cycle, or over several. A cyst can form when a follicle fails to ovulate and continues growing. There's also a luteal cyst, which can sometimes cause symptoms when the corpus luteum bleeds into its capsule or into the pelvic cavity. The pain associated with this tends to be acute and to resolve after twenty-four hours. These are both examples of physiological cysts, which are the most common type of ovarian cyst and tend to resolve on their own, although sometimes they may need intervention. However, pathological cysts – which include dermoid cysts (as Gabby had) – can cause more persistent and significant symptoms.

Gabby was a perfectionist, a solicitor in a big firm, who was putting in regular 12–14-hour days. She appeared to have her life under full control but, on deeper questioning, it became clear that her drive came from her difficult relationship with her father. He was a barrister and was her constant critic.

Gabby had lost her mother when she was a teenager, but rather than being able to grieve with those close to her, she had had to step into the matriarchal role, looking after her siblings. From this point on, she became driven by a need to prove that she was capable and that others could depend on her. But she felt she could never express the resentment and unfairness she experienced over this.

As an adult, Gabby found it hard to be intimate with herself or a partner, unable to reconcile her high-powered work persona with her other needs, which seemed inappropriate and selfish. She felt trapped in a job with constant pressure to climb the ladder. Even when her cyst was painful, she continued to put in long hours. She also felt trapped by anger towards her dad and her boss, both of whom were domineering; and, most of all, towards herself for falling victim to the financial gains of a job that she didn't find fulfilling and that kept her disconnected from herself.

Gabby went on to have surgery to remove the cyst. Alongside this, she also did some deep healing in her relationship with her father and herself, in order to reduce the risk of a recurrence. She learned to be more honest and connected with herself and, soon afterwards, left her job to find one that was more aligned with her authentic self.

I have seen, over and over again, how in cases like Connie's and Gabby's, doing TCP can help with symptoms. For ovarian health, it's vital that you have the space, time and platform to be able to release your frustration and anger as well as to speak your mind and truth, in order to channel them towards something good or creative.

You may not have been given the best circumstances in life, but you have the capacity to invest in cultivating new experiences and creating new environments both inside and outside your body, which will become the emotional and physical seeds of your future, your health and your fertility, as well as the health of any future baby.

> ## PCOS AND EATING DISORDERS
>
> Women with PCOS have a higher rate of disordered eating. It's often assumed this is a result of PCOS, but it may be that disordered eating is a trigger, causing epigenetic changes that lead to PCOS. We know that both PCOS and eating disorders are associated with being a high achiever and/or a perfectionist. The emotional underpinnings of both are similar: girls and young women whose lives can feel full of chaos or turmoil, and who need to gain a sense of control over what can feel overwhelming. The outward sign of this is by controlling food and/or weight. But the inner sign may be a multitude of repressed emotions, leading to PCOS. The HPG axis, which is the main method of communication between the brain and the reproductive organs, can become oversensitized as a result of mental and physical stress, and that can lead to epigenetic changes, which in turn lead to PCOS.

Journaling prompts for ovarian conditions

* Do you believe that success only comes from hard work and challenges?

* Do you have difficulty accepting your attractiveness as a woman?

* Do you have negative associations with being a woman?

* Were there issues of abandonment or other trauma that affected the women in your lineage?

❋ Have you felt under pressure to accept more masculine roles in your life?

❋ Do you feel under pressure to appear strong and capable all the time?

❋ What was your relationship like with your mother and father?

❋ Did you ever feel a sense of rejection or disappointment from either of them?

❋ How were the women in your lineage treated by men?

❋ Is there a history of abuse either with yourself or with other women in your lineage?

❋ What is your relationship like with men?

❋ How do you feel about expressing your sexual needs?

❋ Are there repeating patterns of hostility and abuse in your relationships?

❋ Do you find it hard accepting that something could come to you with ease and have come to feel more comfortable and familiar with facing challenges or difficulties instead?

TCP advice for ovarian disease

In addition to TCP, here are some areas to focus on for ovarian conditions:

Nutrition

❋ **Eat foods rich in zinc**: organic grass-fed meat, shellfish, legumes, squash, pumpkin and sesame seeds, cashews, almonds, eggs and dark chocolate, for its antioxidant and anti-inflammatory properties.

✳ **Eat more vitamin C-rich foods**, such as strawberries, oranges, red peppers and broccoli, as this may help to regulate the activity of genes needed for follicle development.

✳ **Help to support the liver and its natural detoxification processes** by incorporating lemon juice and bitter greens, such as dandelion, endive and radicchio. Or use liver-supporting herbs, such as dandelion root, milk thistle and turmeric. Remember: once you're pregnant, consult a doctor regarding the use of herbs.

✳ **Add seaweed to your diet to increase the amount of iodine** if you are thyroid-deficient, as well as Brazil nuts that contain selenium.

✳ **Incorporate broccoli and leafy greens into your diet** as they contain diindolylmethane, which may help the body remove excess oestrogen.

✳ **Supplement with healthy fats like Omega 3**, to support the probiotic population in the gut that helps to keep a natural balance in hormones and neurotransmitters.

✳ **Keep well hydrated with water**, consume plenty of fibre and incorporate aloe-vera juice to treat chronic constipation, which can prevent adequate absorption of nutrients and encourage the storage of fat and excess nutrients.

✳ **Reduce oxidative stress** by supplementing with glutathione, vitamin C and CoQ10.

✳ **Consume lots of lean protein** to provide raw materials for hormone and neurotransmitter production.

✳ **Supplementing with N-acetyl cysteine (NAC)** can improve mitochondrial function, repair damaged cells and reduce inflammation.

❋ **Eat food-sourced vitamin A (not synthetic versions)** in asparagus, carrots, broccoli and kale, which may help to reduce the risk of ovarian cancer.

Exercise

❋ **Increase your metabolism through regular cardiovascular exercise,** and reduce fat stores to increase your body's natural ability to release oestrogenic chemicals that are trapped in adipose cells.

❋ **Mitochondrial fatigue can lead to tiredness after exercise,** so preserving and building muscle mass as you age is important, to counteract some of this effect.

❋ **If you have a large ovarian cyst,** ask your doctor for specific advice about exercise, because a strenuous workout might be painful and may possibly lead to ovarian torsion (twisting).

Stress

❋ **Our chakra system is closely related to our endocrine glands** and these two systems work closely in tandem. The chakra system is also supported by the meridian system, which orchestrates the flow of energy between chakras and is heavily influenced by emotions. We require regular detoxification of our emotions for all of this to run smoothly. Incorporate the meditations set out in the 12-week plan, covering all of the seven different chakras.

❋ **Refined sugar, distorted fats, preservatives, pesticides and alcohol** can increase intestinal permeability, disturb the microbiome and create hyperarousal, which increases stress and anxiety, so keeping these to a minimum in your diet is important.

✳ **Get seven to nine hours of sleep each night**, as studies show that getting less can lead to obesity and insulin resistance by reducing the amount of fat-busting hormones, such as growth hormone, leptin and melatonin.

✳ **Vitamin D appears to be able to regulate sleep** by acting on the part of the brain that's in charge of our hormones, and the brainstem. Studies have also shown that low vitamin D can increase the perception of pain in the body, leading to insomnia.

✳ **Make time each day to do something creative for you**, because the ovaries are associated with being a creative centre in the body. This will not only bring pleasure, but will help with stress, too.

✳ **Massage can help to relieve tension**, and acupuncture can help to regulate ovulation.

Relationships

✳ **Commit to cultivating a better relationship with yourself and your body**: regularly stop and pay attention to how your body feels. Tune into what it needs, whether it's to go to the loo, rest or express an emotion. When a sensation arises, if you can, stop what you're doing, lie down and breathe and lean into the feeling. If there is pain, attempt to see if you can trace the trigger.

✳ **Notice how certain people in your life make you feel**, whether their behaviour triggers specific sensations in your body, and whether this enables you to step into your wholeness and a feeling of being free to be yourself or keeps you stifled and curtailed in your self-expression.

✳ **Pay attention to your inner voice**: if you can become conscious of what's subconscious, then you can reflect on the effect that voice has and focus on changing it.

❊ **Notice if there are parts of you that you dislike or have disowned**: imagine how you'd respond to a loved one who had these same insecurities; say to yourself what you'd say to them. It may be helpful to limit your exposure to media messaging that encourages toxic body beliefs and comparison.

❊ **Clear your emotional energetic residues** with the help of an energetic healer who can help you tap into this, via the chakra and meridian systems. Or use the techniques outlined in the 12-week plan to help.

TCP advice for PCOS

❊ **Remember that food cravings, binge-eating and weight management** are not simply causes, but also effects, of PCOS. A lower-carb diet where any carbs are low-GI (see page 85) will help to improve insulin sensitivity and so reduce androgens. Reduce your consumption of refined grains, such as white rice, corn and wheat.

❊ **Make sure you get enough protein and good fats**, such as Omega 3 (in fish and supplements) and organic virgin coconut oil.

❊ **Eating a mainly plant-based diet** can help to balance blood sugar, support oestrogen metabolism, restore the gut microbiome and increase the body's own detoxification processes.

❊ **Eating regular meals will help too**.

❊ **Good foods to eat**: sesame seeds help reduce androgens; beans and lentils provide inositol, which helps keep blood sugars balanced; broccoli and leafy greens contain diindolylmethane, which helps the body to remove excess oestrogen.

❋ **Reduce or eliminate dairy products** or consider switching from cow-based products to sheep- or goat-based ones. Consider cutting out gluten from your diet too, to see if it helps improve symptoms.

❋ **Eliminate cured processed meats** that contain nitrates, which can increase obesity and diabetes.

❋ **Additional supplements**, such as essential fatty acids (evening primrose or cod-liver oil), saw palmetto and inositol, may help to improve metabolism as well as promoting a healthy hormonal balance.

❋ **Vitamin D can alter AMH signalling, FSH sensitivity, progesterone production and release** that may be needed during normal follicular development. In women with PCOS who are low in vitamin D, supplementing with vitamin D can lower abnormally raised AMH, indicating that the vitamin may improve folliculogenesis.

❋ **Incorporate beans, walnuts, bananas and salmon** to increase natural levels of vitamin B that may help to reduce homocysteine levels and reduce cardiovascular risk.

❋ **Bisphenol A and pesticides can both mimic the action of oestrogen**, and perfluorooctanoate has been found in increased levels in the serum of women with PCOS. Exposure to these substances in products, whether that's in contaminated food or toiletries used pre-natally and post-natally, can influence the development of PCOS in the baby.

❋ **If you are overweight**, regular exercise will not only help to manage your overall BMI, but will also help to reduce androgen levels, improve your sensitivity to insulin, help to restore more regular ovulation and increase lean muscle mass. Just a 5 per cent reduction in weight in those with a high BMI can help to restore normal ovulation.

❋ **If you are not overweight**, there is a subtype of PCOS where women can have a low or normal BMI. Be cautious with the amount of exercise you do. If you have this form of PCOS, excessive exercise will increase stress, activating the HPA axis and stimulating the adrenal glands to produce even more androgens, which will set off all the vicious cycles of PCOS. Resistance training, in particular, has been shown to be more effective in this type of PCOS.

❋ **Adding resistance training** helps to reduce fat around the abdominal organs, reduce androgen levels, improve menstrual irregularities and increase lean muscle mass.

❋ **Spend at least fifteen minutes a day in natural sunlight**, to trigger a host of hormonal and enzymatic reactions that maintain optimal weight, and which stimulate the pineal gland to secrete melatonin at night. This also produces vitamin D, which we need in order to absorb calcium, which in turn is needed to produce stomach acid. If there isn't enough stomach acid, then food can't be digested correctly, so the brain sends out signals that encourage further eating in order to compensate and can contribute to obesity.

❋ **Yoga has been shown** to reduce imbalances in the autonomic nervous system, reduce cortisol, reduce inflammation, while raising serotonin and dopamine that help to stabilize mood. Yoga also raises nitric oxide and glutathione, helping to deliver more blood flow to muscles and organs.

❋ **Regular exercise helps** to reset the HPA axis, turn off the FTO (fat mass and obesity-associated) gene, which carries a risk of obesity and diabetes, and increase sensitivity to insulin. Make sure exercise is kept in moderation, though, as too much can interfere with the HPG axis and lead to absent ovulation and menstruation.

❊ **Exercise also improves methylation**, which influences epigenetic patterns and allows the muscles to soak up sugar more efficiently, reducing the risk of diabetes.

❊ **Exercise can help to switch on longevity genes** and release the hormone irisin, which turns white fat into brown fat, which helps to absorb sugar and reduces insulin resistance.

CHAPTER 18

TCP for Fallopian-tube conditions

‖‖‖

Melanie started trying to conceive with her husband, Simon, when she was thirty-two. After two years of trying she had investigations, including a laparoscopy. The operation found evidence that Melanie had had chlamydia and pelvic inflammatory disease (PID), which had affected both of her Fallopian tubes, which were scarred. Their doctor suggested that Melanie could either have an operation to have her tubes repaired (although he was clear that this was not always successful) or could proceed to IVF. Melanie decided to attempt the repair, as the couple were keen to try to conceive naturally in the first instance.

After the repair, the couple tried again for a year, but still Melanie didn't get pregnant. She went for a dye test (hysterosalpingography or HSG), which found that both of her Fallopian tubes were patent (open) as a result of the previously successful operation. However, as the couple had tried to become pregnant for three years by then, they decided to get on the list to receive IVF.

When I asked Melanie about her past, it became clear there were several important issues affecting her. The relationship she had with both her parents was difficult. Her mother was a domineering figure who was still trying to control Melanie, just as she had in childhood, imposing her views, meaning that Melanie often felt under pressure to please her. Her mother had had several affairs and eventually separated from Melanie's father. As a result, Melanie shouldered disproportionate responsibilities from early on in her life, where stress and trauma were projected onto her, which affected her self-esteem. She realized that her previous intimate relationships had allowed her to regain a sense of worthiness and control – something that she had struggled to find within herself as a result of earlier-life trauma.

Therapy allowed Melanie to gradually rebuild and repair her relationship with her mother and father. She also had regular acupuncture and began to eat healthily. It was during this time that she became pregnant naturally and conceived her son. She gave birth to a healthy baby boy. Two years later, when the couple tried for a second child, Melanie conceived naturally again, but had an ectopic pregnancy. She underwent a salpingectomy to remove the affected Fallopian tube. Realizing the importance of her emotions, she allowed herself to grieve the loss of her baby and to process the feelings that came up in her. Soon after this, she conceived her second son naturally.

The Fallopian tubes extend around 10–12cm from each side of the womb, opening near the ovaries. They form the bridge between the ovulated egg and the womb. But Fallopian tubes are not simply passive mechanical pipes. One of their jobs is to collect the egg from the ovary. Usually this is done by the Fallopian tube on the same side as the ovary that has ovulated. However, in some circumstances the tube on the opposite side can reach across to collect the ovulated egg.

The coming together of the egg and sperm is an amazing feat of engineering, requiring a complex interaction of hormonal, neurological and epigenetic factors. Fallopian tubes play a big part in facilitating fertilization, and indeed whether a pregnancy happens at all. They not only capture eggs and provide an environment for that egg, but also store and activate sperm. Just as the cells in the lining of the womb respond to cyclical hormones, so the cells lining the tubes do too. In fact the Fallopian tubes are exposed to a high concentration of hormones from the ovaries because they absorb the hormone-rich follicular fluid from the ovulated follicles. These hormones prompt the tubes to contract in a specific way so that the egg and sperm meet in the right place.

The tubes are also the first environment of a potential new pregnancy, helping to keep the embryo nourished during its first few days.

Their cells secrete growth factors, cytokines and other factors that support the development of the embryo.

Finally, the Fallopian tubes propel the embryo via finely orchestrated contractions to the uterus, enabling implantation in the correct place. This journey takes around five days. The contractions also help to reduce the chance of more than one sperm fertilizing an egg. Fallopian tubes are fragile and can easily be damaged: both inflammation and infection – most commonly PID – can lead to adhesions that stop them working properly. Up to 80 per cent of women with endometriosis have some form of scarring seen across their Fallopian tubes at laparoscopy (keyhole surgery).

Fallopian tubes and the epigenome

The epigenome of the Fallopian tubes influences everything from the microbial environment, fertilization, the propulsion of tubal fluid and embryos, and their direction of travel, as well as directing where implantation takes place.

The Fallopian tube and its microenvironment provide an ideal set of conditions for early embryo development. But epigenetic changes in genes and proteins of the Fallopian tube can lead to alterations in the environment and thus change the gene expression of the developing embryo. They can lead to abnormalities with fertilization and implantation too. When these epigenetic changes affect the microbiome, they can predispose the woman to conditions such as PID and inflammation.

TCP pillars may help optimize Fallopian function via the epigenome. The changes made at this level may be able to have an indirect influence on tubal contractions, as explained above, and the tubal fluid produced by the cells that line the Fallopian tubes. For example, patients with endometriosis have been shown to have more inflammatory mediators in this fluid, which may negatively impact on fertilization. An abnormal epigenetic environment in the Fallopian tubes has also been implicated in ovarian cancer; there is research looking into this.

In 2005 researchers identified proteins on the surface of sperm and eggs that are essential for one to fuse with the other. The sperm's binding protein is called Izumo 1, after a Japanese marriage shrine. And the egg's binding protein is called Juno, after the Roman goddess of marriage and fertility. The Juno–Izumo interaction – a harmonious balance between giving and receiving – is a vital part of fertilization. And it's likely to be controlled by various epigenetic factors, some of which could have an emotional basis. The Fallopian tubes have receptors to stress hormones – specifically the CRH (corticotrophin-releasing hormone) receptor, which suggests that the tubes' function is affected by our emotional and mental state (see Chapter 8). Studies have shown that CRH and other stress hormones can impair embryo development in the Fallopian tubes by causing oxidative stress to the cells of the tubes; this suggests one way in which a very early pregnancy may be vulnerable to the impact of stress. As we'll see, CRH is important for other reasons too, including influencing implantation and very possibly it has a role in preventing ectopic pregnancy.

Factors in ectopic pregnancy

An ectopic pregnancy is when an embryo implants in the wrong place – usually in a Fallopian tube, although it can be elsewhere in the pelvis or abdomen. One of the most common causes is a previous untreated pelvic infection leading to PID. As well as pain and having to go to hospital for treatment, an ectopic pregnancy can be very distressing (see Chapter 12 for more on this) because a pregnancy anywhere outside the womb is not viable. It can often be treated with medication, but sometimes the woman will need surgery to remove the Fallopian tube, because it can be life-threatening

For the embryo to end up in the right place at the right time is a complicated process. Tubal movement needs to synchronize epigenetically with embryo and endometrial development. For example, the CRH receptor has a role in early embryo implantation, affecting whether there are any abnormalities with this. Abnormal expression of the CRH receptor in the Fallopian tubes is associated with ectopic pregnancies, probably due to a change in cell dynamics and blood-vessel formation.

It seems that genes carried by the embryo play a part in this too, in the way they respond to their environment. And coordination of Fallopian-tube contractions as well as follicular-fluid flow is also needed; abnormalities in both can lead to ectopic pregnancies. This is controlled by altered expression of particular genes. It is possible that, by optimizing the epigenetic environment in the tubes and endometrium through the lifestyle advocated by TCP, the risk of ectopic pregnancy may be reduced.

The consciousness of what happens in the Fallopian tubes

When the egg and sperm join together, they undergo not only structural changes, but also a change in consciousness. Women who have conditions affecting their Fallopian tubes that interfere with or prevent fertilization also often have emotional histories that mirror what's happening at the cellular level. That might be a history of an intrusion or breach of boundaries, difficulty standing up for themselves and disempowerment.

CASE STUDY

Sasha was twenty-nine and had been diagnosed with a Fallopian-tube abscess, secondary to a pelvic infection. She'd grown up with a mother who had turned to alcohol to deal with her emotional issues, and a father who had left her and her mother when she was nine. Her mother had told her that her father had been abusive towards her, even while she was pregnant with Sasha.

Sasha wasn't sure she ever wanted to be a parent, as a result of witnessing her parents and their rows, and turned to sex from the age of thirteen to help her find a sense of worthiness and love. Sex helped her to feel validated, but she struggled to impose her own boundaries upon it and, despite not using regular contraception, didn't find herself becoming pregnant over the course of time — something that can be an important sign of fertility being compromised.

She tended to attract men who were verbally abusive and demeaning, and over time, instead of making her feel empowered, the relationships often left her feeling diminished. Sasha told me her diagnosis made her feel resentful of all the times she didn't stand up for herself and her own body, allowing men with whom she was involved to dominate her sense of self. She struggled with her self-worth. In addition, she didn't trust herself to be a good mother, and felt that the abscess she had was a punishment for some of the earlier life decisions she'd made.

Sasha went on to have the Fallopian tube affected by the abscess surgically removed, but an important part of her recovery and preparation for motherhood – which she realized was important to her, after facing the grief of losing one of her Fallopian tubes – was to engage with all her previously unacknowledged emotions through mind–body therapies and counselling. The abscess was a means of bringing up these emotions, to help her regain a sense of power over her own body, as well as establishing a more compassionate relationship with herself.

There are some other typical patterns of behaviour that I've seen in women who have conditions affecting the Fallopian tubes. Like the case studies shared here, they can have a childhood history that was lacking in love, presence, nurturing or protection. And in common with all the other reproductive conditions, the Mother Wound (see page 66) plays a major part too.

As children, they may have been guilt-tripped, emotionally manipulated or driven into compliance. As a consequence, they can often sideline their own needs to fulfil those of others, whether that's a parent or a partner. They take on others' responsibilities and struggle to set personal boundaries. They downplay their own passions or talents through a sense of duty, but this builds resentment inside them, as well as feelings of entrapment, despair and grief over the loss of themselves. They may even have become numb to their feelings, having learned to hide them in order to put others first. And they often carry a burden of pressure from a parental figure or a partner. As a result, they may not be able to connect to a true sense of identity, but instead fulfil the many roles that others expect of them.

Journaling prompts for Fallopian-tube conditions

❋ Do you carry any resentments over being controlled, manipulated or having your dreams curtailed in order to appease someone?

❋ In what areas of your life have you felt you may have sacrificed or self-sabotaged?

❋ What is your relationship with yourself like? Do you feel limited in what you think you can do?

❋ Do you have trouble imposing personal boundaries and/or feel they are under threat or challenged?

❋ Do you feel many of your relationships have an imbalance of power that goes against you?

❋ In what parts of your life have you felt undermined and underappreciated?

❋ What parts of you have you numbed out, to avoid feeling emotional pain from previous circumstances or situations?

TCP advice for Fallopian-tube conditions

Follow the advice in the TCP pillars, Chapter 16 and Chapter 19, customized with these additions:

❋ **Eat immune-boosting foods rich in vitamin C, vitamin E and zinc**, which can help to prevent a recurrence of infections.

❋ **Incorporate garlic into your diet**, as it has strong antibacterial properties.

* **Incorporate organic virgin coconut oil**, which is a saturated fat with antibacterial and antiviral properties that help support the immune system, as well as protecting the nervous system.

* **Try acupuncture or pelvic massage to improve blood and lymph flow in the pelvis.** If you know you have pelvic adhesions, an adjustment by an osteopath or chiropractor may help relieve pelvic tension and assist realignment.

* **Do a castor-oil treatment** (but *not* with acute PID): this will help to invigorate blood flow and the lymphatic system. Lying down, rub castor oil on your stomach, cover it with cling film, then place a towel and then hot-water bottle on top. Relax for twenty minutes.

* **Avoid using the copper IUD**, which has been linked to a higher incidence of PID as well as ectopic pregnancy.

* **Optimize your reproductive microbiome** through the measures described earlier in the book.

* **Stop smoking**, as it negatively impacts on conception in multiple ways. One of them is that nicotine affects Fallopian-tube contractions and the action of the cilia, being associated with a higher risk of PID.

* **Make sure your hands and fingernails are clean before sex (and your partner's are too)**: good hygiene, taking regular exercise and reducing stress increase your blood levels of albumin, a protein that helps deal with infection. Albumin also positively impacts on several hormones, including growth hormone and insulin, as well as helping to eliminate toxins.

* **Untreated vaginal infections** can infect your partner's prostate gland, impact on their sperm and create reinfection — another important reason to get screened and to treat infections in you and your partner.

* **If you've had an ectopic pregnancy**, read Chapter 12.

CHAPTER 19

TCP for conditions of the vulva, vagina and cervix

CASE STUDY

Bianca, forty-one, came to me when she was looking to conceive her second child. She had experienced recurrent miscarriages since the birth of her first child and said she struggled to feel present during sex. She had had treatment to remove abnormal cells on her cervix when she was in her twenties. These kinds of abnormal cells begin as infection with HPV, a common virus that is transmitted sexually and skin-to-skin.

Bianca told me that, growing up, her father was often absent and was unfaithful to her mother. She remembered a lot of arguments, and seeing her mother drink to numb her pain. As a teenager, Bianca turned to smoking, drugs and alcohol too, to numb her feelings of being neglected and not good enough. As an adult, she felt under constant pressure to prove herself, disowning her own needs to please others. She had relationships with toxic men who were never emotionally available. Her ex, the father of her child, had also been unfaithful and abusive, so Bianca had felt unsafe while pregnant, even wondering whether she could carry on with the pregnancy.

She was now with a different partner and had given up her destructive habits, but she was struggling and scared that pregnancy would make her vulnerable again. Tied in with this were fears that it might put her and her partner's relationship under strain, and that she might go back to her previous self-sabotaging behaviours, such as drinking and taking drugs.

Bianca started seeing a therapist to deal with her emotional patterns. She had an open discussion with her partner, who was patient and understanding; he started seeing a therapist too, for his own earlier-life trauma. Bianca committed to reclaiming her reproductive organs and cultivating her own feelings of safety. She and her partner are in the process of trying naturally, and both feel a deep calling to be parents to another child.

One of the most complicated relationships many women have is the one with their own vagina and vulva. Nearly half of women have never discussed their vagina with anyone, due to embarrassment and even shame. Forty per cent of women can't correctly name the vulva. Two-thirds are reluctant to engage in oral sex for fear of this most intimate part of themselves being judged.

It's not unusual that, during a smear test, a woman will apologize for the appearance of her vulva. One-third of women suffer from painful sex; more than half of these women have vaginismus, painful spasmodic tightening of the vagina, which can be activated even by the thought of having something inserted into the vagina. Smear tests can be traumatic and as you'll see later, the vagina, like other reproductive organs, can store memories of this trauma that may have biological consequences. The same can happen during labour: many women hold on to trauma from obstetric examinations or a difficult childbirth experience.

One reason women struggle with this part of their body, and why many don't necessarily seek help, is because it's considered taboo. Perhaps you were told as a child that it was dirty or wrong to touch your genitals? Or, as a woman, you've been shamed for expressing your sexuality? Or you may have taken on board the distorted cultural view that this area needs to be sanitized and disguised, whether through extensive hair removal or using perfumed washes or deodorants? Or even aesthetically corrected? Labiaplasty is now the fastest-growing cosmetic operation; even some prepubescent girls ask to have it.

Our misogynistic modern culture plays a big part in women's bodily disconnect and shame. The vulva was once a revered symbol of the sacred feminine – one that appears in places of worship, from caves to churches (you'll notice as you walk into a church that the arch, or apse, resembles the opening of the vagina; this is no coincidence). This part of a woman's body was there to be worshipped and adored, representing a portal between the spiritual and the material, as well as being a symbol of cosmic creation.

Thousands of years of violations to women's bodies have disconnected them from their innate sacredness. More than a quarter of women worldwide have experienced sexual abuse by the time they're eighteen. But even outside physical assault, often women and girls are verbally abused and shamed over their sexual identities. A woman who expresses her sexuality is seen as impure. Societies continue to judge and control women and their bodies by shaming them, whether it's over the number of their sexual partners or their reproductive choices.

Our current distorted culture, when it comes to women and girls, has literally become ingrained in the reproductive anatomy. One reason this messaging and the beliefs that surround it are so powerful is because the clitoris, vulva, vagina and cervix are neurologically wired directly to the brain. It turns out that ancient Eastern Tantric beliefs were ahead of their time; now we can truly appreciate the wisdom of their belief that the reproductive organs are a means of accessing enlightenment and a shift in consciousness. The clitoris and vagina are connected to the spinal cord via the pudendal nerve, and the cervix via the pelvic nerve – all of them eventually feeding into the brain. But as branches of these two nerves vary in their distribution and concentration, every woman will have her own unique sexual response.

This wiring is also why experiences involving our genitals – both positive and negative, including examinations and smear tests – can create new brain connections of pleasure or trauma. And it's why sex can trigger memories of past trauma or previous abuse too.

There are more than 100 euphemisms in the English language for the vulva and vagina, and most are used in a derogatory way. Even medically, we refer to structures in this area as 'pudendal', a word originating from the Latin *pudere*, meaning 'to be ashamed'. Words hurt. As we've seen earlier in the book, pain can become psychogenic, meaning that the mental source of pain can manifest physically: debasing the vulva and vagina, even just verbally, sends a signal to the woman's brain that she isn't safe. Like any kind of abuse, this can rewire the brain at the level of the amygdala – the emotional centre – and can lead to the same effects as trauma. Abuse, in all its various forms, creates anxiety and fear that can also inhibit genital arousal, causing vaginal dryness and pelvic-floor hypertonicity (stiffening of the pelvic-floor muscles), contributing to the pain of vaginismus.

Painful sex, vaginismus and vulvodynia

If you are someone who suffers from painful sex, it's important to see your doctor as there are a lot of possible physical causes that are correctible, including thrush and irritation; or if the pain is deeper, perhaps ovarian cysts or PID.

But the leading cause of painful sex is vulvodynia (chronic pain in and around the vulva), where the pain has no obvious physical cause and so it's seemingly unexplained. Vulvodynia often includes vaginismus too. It has emotional roots; women who experience it are three times more likely to have had some form of abuse, or to be living with the threat of abuse, compared to those who don't have the condition. In Chapter 5 you learned how abuse can manifest as disease in the body. Numbness, pain, not wanting to have sex and dissociation are all reactions by our bodies to protect us from the emotional trauma that we struggle to face. Seen from this perspective, vaginismus and vulvodynia are the vulva reflecting the same kind of dysregulation as the brain in response to traumatic experiences, becoming sensitized to pain and to memories stored in its cells.

CASE STUDY

Ruth, forty-five, came to see me because she had a cyst in her vulva that kept recurring, despite being drained and then surgically removed. It was causing her pain and stopping sex being pleasurable. Her instinct was that there were recurring emotional patterns behind the cyst. As we explored these issues,

Ruth told me she was the middle child and had never felt good enough. There was generational trauma in her family lineage too, from sexual abuse that had never been openly discussed and was kept taboo. This had led to Ruth having a sense of shame around sex.

She said she'd spent most of her life trying to please others, including her previous partner. He'd been emotionally and physically abusive. Sex became the tool that gave her a sense of power and validation that she didn't feel she got anywhere else. She told me, 'I allowed myself to become a victim, using my vagina as a tool to prove my self-worth and develop a co-dependent relationship with my partner. My childhood beliefs of "being stupid", and an unhealthy coping mechanism of not wanting to make a fuss, trapped me into a loop of inauthenticity and not being able to set boundaries, such as saying no to sex.'

Ruth eventually left the abusive relationship and found a wonderful man who was able to support her as she faced her previous trauma. But she struggled to find sex fulfilling, often experiencing numbness and using sex toys to help her achieve arousal. We discussed how to change the narrative of the relationship between herself and her vulva and vagina, deepening the connection and increasing her ability to connect and be present with the emotions that came up for her.

Ruth said that she wanted to learn to express herself and articulate her needs; she even gave her vulva a name, Nessa. She started being mindful of the words she was using when describing Nessa and developing a much deeper relationship with her, through her work with an intimacy coach. She also spent time masturbating without using sex toys, and cultivating the relationship between herself and her vagina. Her vulval cyst is reducing in size and is no longer painful. Her previous numbness during sex is lessening and she now has a much more fulfilling relationship with her partner, in which she is able to feel safe to be herself fully, express her needs and be held and loved.

The emotional underpinnings of vaginal disease

In energetic terms, the vulva, vagina and cervix are related to the root and sacral chakras. The chakra system is important here because it reacts to environmental cues even before our nervous system, interpreting feelings without us being consciously aware of them. And so dysfunction in a woman's relationship with herself or others will leave an imprint here that can set the foundation for disease.

Explained biologically, the vulva and vagina are highly susceptible to stress. Because this is where the inside meets the outside world, they have a high level of immune activity, and stress can have an epigenetic effect on this because, as we've seen, the immune system is so closely intertwined with many other systems in our body. Trauma and stress can be expressed as hypersensitivity and pain here, or as dissociation and numbness, as happened to Bianca and Ruth. It can also manifest as reduced neurotransmission, blood flow and muscle relaxation. If these epigenetic changes persist, they can lead to changes in cells and tissue in the organ, in the form of disease.

Our emotional environment – the result of thoughts and beliefs we've internalized from the world around us – influences our personality, and that affects the expression of our genes. Any form of coercion, manipulation or abuse, as well as resentment towards the coercers or abusers, can be stored in the vagina and cervix. Loss, rejection or abandonment can all leave lasting legacies on the genitals too. A study showed that stress and a feeling of hopelessness triggered by an abusive relationship are contributing factors to cervical disease.

Women with issues affecting the vagina, vulva or cervix have some typical personality traits they share: putting others above themselves, conforming to a 'good girl' or 'good partner' image, and struggling to impose boundaries. This can lead to women sexually shutting down or having multiple sexual partners who don't treat them respectfully. Women who have had negative experiences related to their sexuality or genitalia often struggle with intimacy and expressing the fullness of their sexual selves, even in safe and loving relationships.

Women who can't have sex due to pain, vulvodynia or vaginismus can end up having IVF to conceive, and sometimes this can be the right treatment. But having a condition related to this area is also an opportunity to look at the deeper issues behind it and treat it. This can enable a couple to conceive naturally and improve the relationship with each other and with themselves. Most importantly of all, it can allow healing. This was the case with a patient called Stephanie, who while growing up only ever heard her father using degrading and abusive words to describe women – many of them related to a woman's genitalia. She developed vaginismus and found it difficult to have sex, as well as having issues with her self-esteem and self-worth. Investing time with a therapist enabled her to trace the roots of the trauma she had internalized and to work through this, to help heal the relationship with herself and her ability to have pleasurable sex. Remember that, as you've learned, unresolved trauma can be inherited and acquired. So identifying and treating the issues leading to vulvodynia or vaginismus is important for well-being as well as conception.

If we don't establish our own important relationship with our vulvas and vaginas early in life before sexual encounters begin, we'll continue to accept other people's opinions and desires as our own, without ever appreciating the uniqueness of our anatomy and how powerful it is.

As we discussed in Chapter 5, we can heal by looking into the emotional pain of the past and re-establishing a healthy relationship with our bodies and our nervous systems, perhaps with the help of a therapist. But the most important thing we can do is learn to love our genitals. Treating any conditions of the vagina and/or vulva involves re-establishing a loving relationship with ourselves and feeling safe in our body.

When we develop greater capacities for general pleasure, not only do we start to have better and more powerful sex, but we also unleash a powerful creative force within ourselves, capable of healing and alchemizing many previously unhealthy experiences. When we prioritize our sexual well-being, many aspects of our health and general life can improve, as well as the relationship we have with ourselves, our partners and all those around us. This leads us to greater self-awareness, evolution and expression – to be who we really are and to own it.

Journaling prompts for conditions related to the vagina

* What was the relationship like between you and your mother? (Refer to the section on the Mother Wound on page 66 for help on reflecting on this subject.)

* What is your general relationship like with men, including your father?

* Is there a pattern of abuse or denigration that affects the female bloodline, including you?

* Do you have difficulty expressing boundaries and, if so, why?

* How do you feel about giving birth and being pregnant?

* Are there any fears or traumas tied in with this?

* How has sex in the past made you feel?

* How have previous sexual partners referred to and treated your genitalia?

* Have your relationships made you feel disempowered or empowered?

* How do you refer to your genitalia, and what sort of relationship have you cultivated with your vulva and vagina over the years?

TCP advice for vaginal, vulval and cervical conditions

In addition to TCP, here are some areas to focus on for vaginal, vulval and cervical conditions:

Nutrition

* **Eliminate pro-inflammatory foods**, such as those that are fried or processed, as this may help to alleviate pain associated with vulvodynia.

❋ **Support the vaginal microflora by eating probiotic (fermented) foods** (yoghurt, kefir, fermented pickles, sauerkraut) **and prebiotic foods** (vegetables and fruit, as well as wholegrains).

❋ **Take cranberry supplements and pure (sugar-free) cranberry juice**: these can help to balance vaginal pH levels and so reduce UTIs and other infections.

❋ **Eat more apples**: they contain the phytoestrogen phloridzin, which can help to stimulate vaginal blood flow and lubrication.

❋ **Eat more soy**, which can help with low oestrogen and improve tone and blood flow to the vagina. *Note*: opt for minimally processed soy foods, such as tofu, edamame, tempeh and miso.

❋ **If you have cervical disease, diet is especially important**: an inflammatory diet, such as one that is high in trans fats and refined sugar, has been associated with a greater risk of cervical dysplasia. But a Mediterranean-style diet rich in antioxidants and anti-inflammatories can have beneficial effects in preventing progression to cancer, and some of this may be due to its positive effects on the microbiome too. Make sure you're getting enough antioxidant vitamins A and C. The oral contraceptive pill has been linked with a slightly higher risk of cervical cancer, so if that refers to you, make sure you're supporting your nutritional needs.

Exercise

❋ **Try Kegel exercises, repeating them ten to fifteen times, three times a day**: exercising the pelvic floor can help to support the system of muscles that protect the pelvic organs, as well as improving vaginal health.

❋ **Try yoga, Pilates and core exercises** to improve your posture. It will also improve your pelvic-floor strength.

❋ **Don't cycle or do spinning classes** if you suffer from recurrent thrush, cystitis or vulvodynia, because the bicycle seat can cause localized inflammation and irritation.

❋ **Consider seeing a pelvic physical therapist** if you have any incontinence or prolapse. Treatment has been shown to improve libido and sexual function, as well as reducing pain during sex.

Toxin-free tips

❋ **Clean your vulva and vagina with water only**; if you want to use soap, make sure it's natural and pH-balanced. Perfumed and synthetic soaps, gels, oils, sprays, antiseptics or deodorants are not only unnecessary, but can be harmful. Avoid using bubble baths and talc too. Celebrate your natural pheromone smell – it's a part of what makes you *you* and also has on important role when it comes to conception.

❋ **Wear loose, natural fibre underwear** that doesn't rub.

❋ **Consider keeping your pubic hair**, although that's a personal preference; it's there to help reduce friction and sweating.

❋ **Consider getting STD tests done together with a partner** before you start being sexually active with them (you can do this later, too, but it's better done at the start before any potential exposure). Until you're in a committed relationship, practise safe sex. Having an STD causes reproductive-tract inflammation, which increases the chance of further STDs, and the effects can be cumulative.

❋ **Wipe from the front to the back**, and don't have vaginal intercourse after anal intercourse unless you've washed in between.

❋ **Steer clear of unnecessary antibiotics**: taking multiple courses of antibiotics to treat recurrent bacterial vaginosis may damage your microbiome. Discuss this with your doctor, as it may be treatable with vaginal probiotic suppositories.

❋ **If you use a sex toy, choose one made from medical-grade silicone or natural materials** rather than plastic, and clean it after each use.

❋ **A UTI can indicate vaginal infection that's crossed over into the urethra, so treating it is important.** Many women can end up getting UTIs after intercourse. Washing after sex can help to reduce the risk. What may also be helpful is not totally emptying your bladder before sex, so that the bladder can act as a buffer and reduce the friction that may lead to infections.

Relationships

❋ **Refer to your vulva and vagina in honouring, deeply appreciative terms each time you speak about them,** and even consider writing them a letter to express your love for them. Speaking and articulating words of compassion and honour to your vulva and vagina may sound silly, but the vagina has a direct neurological connection to the brain and words have power, so it will help to counter the effect of any negative and degrading words, as will self-stroking and caressing this part of yourself.

❋ **Practise appreciation and acceptance while looking at your vagina and vulva with a hand-mirror;** this is also a good time to look for any changes, discoloration, redness or soreness.

❋ **Chat with your close girlfriends about things you might normally find embarrassing;** when you do this with people you trust, it can help you to feel secure and safe, and allows you to realize how many women have the same hang-ups, but feel like the only one affected.

✻ **Make sure you attend your smear test** and speak to
   your nurse or doctor about what they can do to make this
   easier for you, if you struggle with it. Bring a friend as an
   ambassador, if that helps. After your smear, honour yourself
   with a small celebration such as flowers, to create a positive
   association with the procedure.

✻ **Stretch, stroke and massage your vagina to help make
   it supple and deepen your connection**: Pilates, yoga and
   Kegel exercises can help to restore normal blood flow and
   improve sensation, along with this.

✻ **Reclaiming this part of our bodies** can often be associated
   with excavating old trauma and wounds, and an
   experienced counsellor or therapist may be invaluable
   here. Do seek help, as this is a really important part of your
   personal evolution.

✻ **Physiotherapy, chiropractic and osteopathy** may all
   be beneficial in relieving the muscle tension and spasm
   associated with vaginismus. Biofeedback that involves
   relaxing and rehabilitating the pelvic floor to re-establish
   normal connections with the vagina and lessen the pain, plus
   TENS treatment (transcutaneous electrical nerve stimulation)
   that uses a low-volt electrical current, may also help.

Conclusion

You may be at the beginning of your conception journey or you may have found yourself struggling for a while. Wherever you are in your journey, this book is here to help guide you through what can be a confusing and uncertain time. It's my sincerest desire to support you to make the lasting changes that will determine the course of your health and that of any children you have for years to come. I hope that by reading this book you have been able to see how much there is that you can do to help yourself, and how it's directly accessible to anyone willing to view their health and fertility through a different lens.

The process of conceiving is often one of healing, which ultimately brings us home to ourselves and restores the power into our hands. My clients following the principles of TCP find that, over time, many other areas of their lives start flourishing too. When we create, we do so in all aspects of our lives. This is what it means to be fertile. It isn't solely about creating another human being, but also about opening ourselves up to the possibility of creating a whole new version of ourselves. This involves becoming conscious of all the different elements that make up our health, from the food we eat, to the environment we expose ourselves to and the thoughts we ruminate over each day. We develop an awareness of the events that have shaped who we are now and become ready to step onto a path of self-evolution, which involves becoming curious about the challenges we face and being open to transforming them.

Conceiving a child is when spirit and science come together, and both of these realms need to be addressed. The journey towards conception starts much earlier than most people presume it does. It goes all the way back to our childhoods and our own personal experiences, which shape who we become. When we do the work that is necessary to become healthier, we also heal any unhealthy generational patterns that have been handed down to us and change the trajectory for our children.

My hope is that this book will encourage a conversation about fertility. The chances are that women in your family, your friends, your colleagues and even the person next to you in the supermarket aisle may be affected by problems in conceiving, but may not feel there are many others out there who are also suffering. The more we share and invite conversations, the more we can stop people going through this in silence and failing to seek the help they need. Whether you choose to keep this book private for yourself or share it with your partner, friends and wider community, I really hope it finds its way into the hands of all of those who need it and changes their lives for the better. I love hearing about each individual path to parenthood, and if you use this book to assist you, please consider sharing on social media with #TheConceptionPlan. Let's start the conversation together and promote a more holistic and inclusive approach to fertility and health.

Although following The Conception Plan will improve your health and optimize your chances of conceiving, there may be instances when this – along with any conventional treatment – does not result in you becoming a parent. It can often feel that you've somehow failed to live up to others' expectations or fallen short of your own dreams. Dealing with the pain of this is one of the most difficult burdens to carry. But please remember, on the other side of it is a person who is wiser, stronger, more resilient and empowered, through the process of their becoming. To be a parent is a blessing, but it isn't a prerequisite to happiness. That can only ever come from within and from realizing that, with or without a child, you are complete and capable of many miracles.

It's my deepest desire that, by reading this book, you become a co-creator of such miracles.

Bibliography

Epigenetics

The Biology of Belief, Bruce Lipton, 2005

The Book You Wish Your Parents Had Read (and Your Children Will Be Glad That You Did), Philippa Perry, 2019

Childhood Disrupted, Donna Jackson Nakazawa, 2015

The Disease Delusion, Jeffrey Bland, 2014

The Epigenetics Revolution, Nessa Carey, 2011

The Longevity Project, Howard Friedman and Leslie Martin, 2012

The Master Builder, Alfonso Martinez Arias, 2023

The Telomere Effect, Dr Elizabeth Blackburn, 2017

What Happened to You?, Bruce Perry and Oprah Winfrey, 2021

What's Going On in There?, Lise Eliot, 1999

'The critical impact of early cellular environment on neuronal development', *Preventative Medicine*, Levitt et al., 1998

'Dads pass on more than genetics in their sperm', smithsonianmag.com, Wu, 2018

'Early experiences can alter gene expression and affect long-term development', *National Scientific Council on the Developing Child*, Harvard University, 2010

'Epigenetics, the misunderstood science that could shed new light on ageing', *The Guardian*, Oct. 2021

'Exploring the epigenetics of resilience', *Nature Genetics*, Dajani, 2022

'Exploring the evidence for epigenetic regulation of environmental influences on child health across generations', *Community Biology*, Breton et al., 2021

'First evidence of how parents' lives could change children's DNA', *New Scientist*, 2015

'Gene-edited butterfly mutants reveal secrets of ancient "junk" DNA', *SciTech Daily*, 2022

'How chronic stress is harming our DNA', *Monitor on Psychology*, 2014

'Neuroendocrine and immune markers of maternal stress during pregnancy and infant cognitive development', *Developmental Psychobioliogy*, Nazzari et al., 2020

'The role of epigenetics in psychological resilience', *The Lancet Psychiatry*, Smeeth et al., 2021

'So called junk DNA – Genetic "Dark Matter" – is actually critical to survival in mammals', University of California, Berkeley, Oct. 2021

Mind–Body

The Biological Mind, Alan Jasanoff, 2018

The Brain That Changes Itself, Norman Doidge, 2007

How Emotions Are Made, Lisa Feldman Barrett, 2017

Living in a Mindful Universe, Dr Eben Alexander, 2017

Molecular Biology of the Cell, Bruce Alberts, 2022

Super Brain, Deepak Chopra and Rudolph Tanzi, 2012

Vibrational Medicine, Richard Gerber, 2001

'Bioenergetics adaptations and redox homeostasis in pregnancy and related disorders', *Molecular and Cellular Biochemistry*, Sanchez-Aranguren et al., 2021

'Depletion of oocyte dynamin-relayed protein 1 shows maternal-effect abnormalities in embryonic development', *Science Advances*, Adhikari et al., 2022

'Epigenetic control of mitochondrial function in the vasculature', *Frontiers in Cardiovascular Medicine*, Mohammed et al., 2020

'Feto-maternal microchimerism: Memories from pregnancy', *Science Direct*, Comitre-Mariano et al., 2022

'Healing touch and fertility: a case report', *Journal of Perinatal Education*, Kissinger et al., 2006

'The heart's electromagnetic field is your superpower', *Psychology Today*, 2020

'Imaginal cells, metamorphosis and emergence', davependle.medium.com, Pendle, 2020

'Microchimerism: how pregnancy . . .', aeon.co, Rowland, 2018

'Ozone and pulsed electromagnetic field therapies improve endometrial lining thickness in frozen embryo transfer cycles', *Medicine*, Merhi et al., 2019

Emotions and Energies

Cure, Jo Marchant, 2016

The Emotion Code, Bradley Nelson, 2007

Lost Connections, Johann Hari, 2018

Meta Human, Deepak Chopra, 2020

Neurodharma, Rick Hanson, 2020

Permission to Feel, Marc Brackett, 2019

The Power of Awakening, Wayne Dyer, 2020

The Power of Now, Eckhart Tolle, 1997

A Radical Awakening, Dr Shefali, 2021

Real Change, Sharon Salzberg, 2020

The Untethered Soul, Michael Singer, 2007

Why Woo-Woo Works, David Hamilton, 2020

'Pregnancy or psychological outcomes of psychotherapy interventions for infertility: a meta-analysis', *Frontiers in Psychology*, Zhou et al., 2021

Infertility

'The comparison of depression and anxiety between fertile and infertile couples: a meta-analysis study', *International Journal of Reproductive BioMedicine*, Fallahzadeh et al., 2019

'Diagnosis and treatment of luteal phase deficiency: a committee opinion', *ASRM*, 2021

'Effects of reproductive history on symptoms of menopause: a brief report', *Menopause*, Nelson et al., 2012

'Emotional aspects of infertility', *Fertility and Sterility*, Seibel et al., 1982

'Genetics and epigenetics of infertility and treatments on outcomes', *JCEM*, Pisarska et al., 2019

'The lasting trauma of infertility', *The New York Times*, Townsend, 2019

'Lifestyle factors and reproductive health: taking control of your fertility', *Reproductive Biology and Endocrinology*, Sharma et al., 2013

'Mini-review on the possible interconnections between the gut-brain axis and the infertility-related neuropsychiatric comorbidities', *Brain Science*, Simionescu et al., 2020

'Physiological aspects of female fertility: role of the environment, modern lifestyle, and genetics', *Physiological Reviews*, Hart et al., 2016

Trauma

Becoming Attached, Robert Karen, 1994

The Body Keeps the Score, Bessel van der Kolk, 2014

The Brain's Way of Healing, Norman Doidge, 2015

How to Do the Work, Nicole LePera, 2021

It Didn't Start with You, Mark Wolynn, 2016

Mindsight, Daniel Siegel, 2010

Mother in the Mother, Pippa Grace, 2019

The Mother Wound, Bethany Webster, 2021

My Grandmother's Hands, Resmaa Menakem, 2017

The Myth of Normal, Gabor Maté, 2022

The Myth of Sanity, Martha Stout, 2001

Raising a Secure Child, Kent Hoffman, Glen Cooper and Bert Powell with Christine Benton, 2017

What Happened To You?, Bruce Perry and Oprah Winfrey, 2021

When the Body Says No, Gabor Maté, 2003

Why Love Matters, Sue Gerhardt, 2004

Widen the Window, Elizabeth Stanley, 2019

'Adverse childhood event experiences, fertility difficulties and menstrual cycle characteristics', *Journal of Psychosomatic Obstetrics and Gynaecology*, Jacobs et al., 2015

'Biological ageing in childhood and adolescence following experiences of threat and deprivation: a systematic review and meta-analysis', *Psychological Bulletin*, McLaughlin et al., 2020

'The biological effect of trauma', *Complex Psychiatry*, Dalvie et al., 2021

'Black–White differences in hysterectomy prevalence: the CARDIA study', *American Journal of Public Health*, Bower et al., 2009

'Can the legacy of trauma be passed down the generations?', BBC Future, 2019

'Early life abuse and risk of endometriosis', *Human Reproduction*, Harris et al., 2018

'Experiencing childhood trauma makes body and brain age faster', American Psychological Association, 2020

'No one talks about the trauma of precocious puberty', medium.com, Bedford, 2020

'Research on central sensitization of endometriosis-associated brain: a systematic review', *Journal of Pain Research*, Zheng et al., 2019

'Trauma during childhood triples the risk of suffering a serious mental disorder in adulthood', *European Archives of Psychiatry and Clinical Neuroscience*, Amann et al., 2022

Nutrition

Animal, Vegetable, Miracle, Barbara Kingsolver with Steven Hopp and Camille Kingsolver, 2007

Deep Nutrition, Catherine and Luke Shanahan, 2008

Eat to Beat Disease, William Li, 2019

Savor, Thuch Nhat Hanh and Lilian Cheung, 2010

'Advanced glycation end products and their relevance in female reproduction', *Human Reproduction*, Merhi et al., 2014

'Decoding a direct dialog between the gut microbiota and the brain', *Neuroscience*, 2022

'Dietary fatty acids affect semen quality', *Andrology*, Esmaeili et al., 2015

'The effect of nutrients and dietary supplements on sperm quality parameters: a systematic review', *Advances in Nutrition*, Salas-Huetos et al., 2018

'Evidence of horizontal gene transfer between human maternal microbiome and infant gut microbiome', *Cell*, Xavier et al., 2022

'Folic acid vs Folate', rootfunctionalmedicine.com, 2022

'Genetically modified food a step closer in England as laws relaxed', *The Guardian*, Sept. 2021

'Genetically modified foods: safety, risks and public concerns – a review', *Journal of Food Science and Technology*, Bawa et al., 2013

'Hormonal birth control depletes your body of key nutrients', naturalwomanhood.org, Stark, 2021

'Human genital tract microbiota: dysbiosis crucial for infertility', *Journal of Endocrinological Investigation*, Venneri et al., 2022

'The impact of food intake and social habits on embryo quality and the likelihood of blastocyst formation', *Reproductive BioMedicine Online*, Braga et al., 2015

'The impact of the gut microbiota on the reproductive and metabolic endocrine system', *Gut Microbes*, Qi et al., 2021

'Nutrition, adult hippocampal neurogenesis and mental health', *British Medical Bulletin*, Zainuddin and Thuret, 2012

'Prenatal learning: Do "pregnancy foods" affect babies' eating habits?', *Parenting Science*, 2022

'Reduction in FSH throughout the menstrual cycle after omega 3 fatty acid supplementation in young normal weight but not obese women', *Reproductive Science*, Bauer et al., 2019

'The role of genital tract microbiome in fertility: a systematic review', *International Journal of Molecular Sciences*, Vitale et al., 2022

'Seafood intake, sexual activity and time to pregnancy', *Journal of Clinical Endocrinology & Metabolism*, Gaskins et al., 2018

'Serum polyunsaturated fatty acids and endometriosis', *Reproductive Science,* Hopeman et al., 2015

www.diabetes.co.uk/food/trans-fats.html
www.naturopathy-uk.com/news/news-cnm-blog/blog/2022/06/27/what-is-the-healthiest-cooking-oil/
www.ncbi.nlm.nih.gov/pmc/articles/PMC6974692/

Exercise

Exercised, Daniel Lieberman, 2020
The Joy of Movement, Kelly McGonigal, 2019
Own the Day, Own Your Life, Aubrey Marcus, 2018

'BMI, physical activity and fecundability in a North American preconception cohort study', *Fertility and Sterility*, McKinnon et al., 2016

'Does exercise affect telomere length?', *Medicina* (Kaunas), Song et al., 2022

'The effect of physical activity on reproductive health outcomes in young women: a systematic review and meta analysis', *Human Reproduction Update*, Mena et al., 2019

'HIIT modulates male factor infertility through anti-inflammatory and anti-oxidative mechanisms', *Cytokine*, Maleki et al., 2020

'Impact of parental exercise on epigenetic modifications inherited by offspring: a systematic review', *Physiological Reports*, Axsom et al., 2019

'Irisin deletion induces a decrease in growth and fertility in mice', *Reproductive Biology and Endocrinology*, Luo et al., 2021

'Maternal physical activity and sedentary behaviour before and during IVF', *Journal of Assisted Reproduction and Genetics*, Soritsa et al., 2020

'Physical exercise: a novel tool to protect mitochondrial health', *Frontiers in Physiology*, Sorriento et al., 2021

'Thermoregulation during pregnancy', *Sports Medicine*, Smallcombe et al., 2021

link.springer.com/article/10.1007/s10815-020-01864-w

Stress

Activate Your Brain, Scott Halford, 2015

Burnout, Emily and Amelia Nagoski, 2019

The Happy Mind, Kevin Horsley and Louis Fourie, 2017

The Inflamed Mind, Edward Bullmore, 2018

The Sleep Revolution, Arianna Huffington, 2016

Sleep Smarter, Shawn Stevenson, 2014

The Stress Code, Richard Sutton, 2018

'Association of MAOA genetic variants and resilience with psychosocial stress: a longitudinal study of Syrian refugees', *PLOS One*, Clukay et al., 2019

'Corticotropin-releasing factor family: a stress hormone-receptor system's emerging role in mediating sex specific signaling', *Cells*, Vuppaladhadiam et al., 2020

'Estrogen receptors and the regulation of the neural stress response', *Neuroendocrinology*, Handa et al., 2012

'Here's how stress can impact your fertility', modernfertility.com, May 2021

'Is it adrenal fatigue? Reassessing the nomenclature of HPA axis dysfunction', ZRT Laboratory, Guilliams, 2017

'Levels of nature and stress response', *Behavioural Science*, Ewert et al., 2018

'Measuring the psychological, biological, and cognitive signatures of profound stress in humanitarian settings: impacts, challenges, and strategies in the field', *Conflict and Health*, Panter-Brick et al., 2020

'The neurobiology of central sensitization', Chronic Pain and Fatigue Research Center, Harte et al., 2022

'Neuron activation near brain base due to stress may lead to infertility in women', *Journal of Neuroscience*, 2020

'Night shift work among women, is it associated with difficulty conceiving a first birth?', *Frontiers in Public Health*, Fernandez et al., 2020

'Overexpression of forebrain CRH during early life increases trauma susceptibility in adulthood', *Neuropsychopharmacology*, Toth et al., 2016

'Pregnenolone steal and the stress effect', amosinstitute.com, Reed, 2022

'Psychological stress and the human immune system: a meta-analytic study of 30 years of inquiry', *Psychological Bulletin*, Segerstrom et al., 2006

'Psychological stress is related to a decrease of serum anti-mullerian hormone level in infertile women', *Reproductive Biology and Endocrinology*, Dong et al., 2017

'Re-assessing the notion of pregnenolone steal', ZRT Laboratory, Guilliams, 2017

'Should fertilization treatment start with reducing stress?', *Human Reproduction*, Campagne, 2006

'Sleep, sleep disturbance and fertility in women', *Sleep Medicine Reviews*, Kloss et al., 2016

'Stress, sex and neural adaptation to a changing environment: mechanisms of neuronal remodeling', *Annals of the New York Academy of Sciences*, McEwan et al., 2010

Toxin-free living

Clean, Alejandro Junger and Amely Greeven, 2009

Count Down, Shanna Swan, 2021

'Epigenetics as a mechanism of linking developmental exposures to long-term toxicity', *Environment International*, Barouki et al., 2018

'Go back to glass bottles to avoid microplastics risk', *The Times*, 2023

'Human health concerns regarding microplastics in the aquatic environment – from marine to food systems', *Science of the total Environment*, Yuan et al., 2022

'Nanoparticles induced potential toxicity on human health: applications, toxicity mechanisms, and evaluation models', *MedComm*, Xuan et al., 2023

'New fears over microplastics in your home', *Daily Mail*, 2021

'Tissue accumulation of microplastics in mice and biomarker responses suggest widespread health risks of exposure', *Scientific Reports*, Deng et al., 2017

'Toxic forever chemicals contaminate indoor air at worrying levels, study finds', *The Guardian*, Aug. 2021

www.bbc.co.uk/news/science-environment-60761972

www.medicalnewstoday.com/articles/230568#1

Sex and relationships

Come As You Are, Emily Nagoski, 2015

How to Be an Adult in Relationships, David Richo, 2002

The Mastery of Love, Don Miguel Ruiz and Janet Mills, 1999

Men Are from Mars, Women Are from Venus, John Gray, 1992

Resurrecting Sex, David Schnarch, 2002

The Science of Orgasm, Barry R. Komisaruk, Carlos Beyer-Flores and Beverly Whipple, 2007

Spiritual Partnership, Gary Zukav, 2009

'Genetic influences on variation in female orgasmic function', *Biology Letters*, Dunn et al., 2005

'HLA-G in human reproduction: aspects of genetics, function and pregnancy complications', *Human Reproduction*, Vauvert et al., 2005

'Semen takes control of females' genes', *Proceedings of the Royal Society B*, Gioti et al., 2012

'Sexual activity, erectile dysfunction, and incident cardiovascular events', *American Journal of Cardiology*, Hall et al., 2010

'Sexual frequency and salivary immunoglobulin A (IgA)', *Psychological Reports*, Charneteski et al., 2004

'Women may ovulate two or three times a month', *British Medical Journal*, Dyer et al., 2003

Male fertility

'A de novo paradigm for male infertility', *Nature Communications*, Veltman, 2022

'The effect of sperm DNA fragmentation on miscarriage rates', *Human Reproduction*, Robinson et al., 2012

'Epigenetics and male reproduction: the consequences of paternal lifestyle on fertility, embryo development and children lifetime health', *Clinical Epigenetics*, Stuppia et al., 2015

'Increased risk of incident of chronic medical conditions in infertile men', *Fertility and Sterility*, Eisenberg et al., 2016

'Is male infertility a forerunner to cancer?', *International Brazilian Journal of Urology*, Burns et al., 2010

'Is the prevalence of Klinefelter syndrome increasing?', *European Journal of Human Genetics*, Morris et al., 2008

'Lifestyle, environmental and additional health factors associated with an increased sperm DNA fragmentation: a systematic review', *Reproductive Biology and Endocrinology*, Szabo et al., 2023

'Paternal age over 50 years decreases assisted reproductive technology success', *Obstetrics and Gynaecology*, Morris et al., 2021

'Rate of de novo mutations and importance of father's age to disease risk', *Nature*, Kong et al., 2012

'Seminal and testicular microbiome and male fertility', *Porto Biomedical Journal*, Brandao et al., 2021

'Temporal trends in sperm count: a systematic review and meta regression analysis', *Human Reproduction Update*, Levine et al., 2017

'What's more, it seems just one copy of the mutation rather than two, is needed to have an adverse impact, meaning that there could be a 50%

chance of this mutation being passed on to a future son and negatively affecting their reproductive capacity', *Nature Communications*, Veltman, 2022

Baby loss

'Altered expression of epigenetic regulators and imprinted genes in human placenta and fetal tissues from second trimester spontaneous pregnancy losses', *Epigenetics*, Vasconcelos et al., 2019

'The association between psychological stress and miscarriage: a systematic review and meta-analysis', *Nature Research*, Qu et al., 2017

'Chromosomally normal miscarriage is associated with vaginal dysbiosis and local inflammation', *BMC Medicine*, Grewal et al., 2022

'Epigenetic cause of miscarriage identified and cured in mice', *Genes and Development*, Inoue et al., 2022

'Epigenetics of recurrent pregnancy loss', *eBioMedicine*, Hocher et al., 2018

'Genetic and epigenetic variations associated with idiopathic recurrent pregnancy loss', *Journal of Assisted Reproduction and Genetics*, Arias-Sosa et al., 2017

'Outcomes of structured psychotherapy for emotional adjustment in a childless couple diagnosed with recurrent pregnancy loss', *Journal of Human Reproductive Science*, Patel et al., 2018

'Potential genetic causes of miscarriage in euploid pregnancies: a systematic review', *Human Reproduction*, Colley et al., 2019

'Pregnancy loss: consequences for mental health', *Frontiers in Global Women's Health*, Cuenca et al., 2022

'Psychological and support interventions to reduce levels of stress, anxiety or depression on women's subsequent pregnancy with a history of miscarriage', *British Medical Journal Open*, Campillo et al., 2017

'Recurrent pregnancy loss: current perspectives', *International Journal of Women's Health*, Hachem et al., 2017

Fertility after thirty-five

Ending Ageing, Aubrey de Grey, 2007

The Longevity Paradox, Steven Gundry, 2019

Super Human, Dave Asprey, 2019

The Telomere Effect, Elizabeth Blackburn and Elissa Epel, 2017

'Advanced maternal age and offspring outcomes: reproductive ageing and counterbalancing period trends', *Population and Development Review*, Barclay et al., 2016

'Advantageous developmental outcomes of advancing paternal age', *Translational Psychiatry*, Janecka et al., 2017

'Fertility and the ageing male', *Reviews in Urology*, Harris et al., 2011

'Having children later in life increases lifespan', *Menopause*, Faubion et al., 2022

'Influence of follicular fluid and cumulus cells on oocyte quality', *Journal of Assisted Reproduction and Genetics*, Broi et al., 2018

'Markers of ovarian reserve as predictors of future fertility', *Fertility and Sterility*, Harris et al., 2022

Assisted reproductive techniques

'Are we overusing IVF?', *British Medical Journal*, Kamphuis et al., 2014

'Epigenetic changes and assisted reproductive technologies', *Epigenetics*, Mani et al., 2020

'Fifteen years of autologous oocyte thaw outcomes from a large university based fertility center', *Fertility and Sterility*, Cascante et al., 2022

'Genes versus children', *Human Reproduction*, Kirkman-Brown, 2020

'Offspring physiology following the use of IVM, IVF and ICSI', *Human Reproduction Update*, Beilby et al., 2023

'Online sperm donation: a survey of the demographic characteristics, motivations, preferences and experiences of sperm donors on a connection website', *Human Reproduction*, Freeman et al., 2016

'Reproductive outcomes from ten years of elective oocyte cryopreservation', *Archives of Gynecology and Obstetrics*, Kasaven et al., 2022

TCP for reproductive conditions

An Elegant Defense, Matt Richtel, 2019

Moody Bitches, Julie Holland, 2015

You Are Your Best Thing, Tarana Burke and Brene Brown, 2021

TCP for womb conditions

Ask Me about My Uterus, Abby Norman, 2018

Period Power, Maisie Hill, 2019

'Different influences of endometriosis and PID on the occurrence of ovarian cancer', *International Journal of Research and Public Health*, Huang et al., 2021

'Effect of psychosocial trauma and stress on sexual dysfunction in women with endometriosis', *Medicine* (Baltimore), Fiala et al., 2021

'Endometrial polyps: pathogenesis, sequelae and treatment', *SAGE*, Nijkang et al., 2019

'How the menstrual cycle changes women's brains – for better', BBC Future, Gorvett, 2018

'The impact of adenomyosis on women's fertility', *Obstetrical and Gynaecological Survey*, Harada et al., 2016

'The importance of a multi-disciplinary approach to the endometriotic patients: the relationship between endometriosis and psychic vulnerability', *Journal of Clinical Medicine*, Carbone et al., 2021

'Infection as a potential cofactor in the genetic-epigenetic pathophysiology of endometriosis: a systematic review', *Facts, Views & Vision in ObGyn*, Koninckx et al., 2019

'The microbiota continuum along the female reproductive tract and its relation to uterine-related diseases', *Nature Communications*, Chen et al., 2017

'Neuroendocrine-immune disequilibrium and endometriosis: an interdisciplinary approach', *Seminars in Immunopathology*, Triverdian et al., 2007

'New opportunities for endometrial health by modifying uterine microbial composition', *Biomolecules*, Molina et al., 2020

'The origin and pathogenesis of endometriosis', *Annual Review of Pathology*, Wang et al., 2020

'Recent advances in uterine fibroid etiology', *Seminars in Reproductive Medicine*, McWilliams et al., 2017

'Steroid hormones regulate genome-wide epigenetic programming and gene transcription in human endometrial cells with marked aberrances in endometriosis', *PLOS Genetics*, Houshadran et al., 2020

'Psychological stress and functional endometrial disorders: update on mechanism insights', *Frontiers in Endocrinology*, Xiang-Wu et al., 2021

'The uterus plays a role in memory', *Medical News Today*, 2018

TCP for ovarian conditions

'Alterations in the intestinal microbiome associated with PCOS affect the clinical phenotype', *Biomedicine & Pharmacotherapy*, Wang et al., 2020

'Chapter Four – Neurotransmitter, neuropeptide and gut peptide profile in PCOS-pathways contributing to the pathophysiology, food intake and psychiatric manifestations of PCOS', *Advances in Clinical Chemistry*, Illie et al., 2020

'Curtailing PCOS', *Paediatric Research*, Feldman Witchel et al., 2019

'Debates regarding lean patients with PCOS: a narrative review', *Journal of Human Reproductive Sciences*, Goyal et al., 2017

'Distinct subtypes of polycystic ovary syndrome with novel genetic associations: an unsupervised, phenotypic clustering analysis', *PLOS Medicine*, Dapas et al., 2020

'Follicle growth and development', GLOWM, Erickson, 2008

'Genetic insights into biological mechanisms governing human ovarian ageing', *Nature*, Ruth, 2021

'Impact of COVID 19 pandemic on the psychosexual functions of healthcare workers', *Journal of Sexual Medicine*, Eroglu et al., 2022

'In search of new therapeutics – molecular aspects of the PCOS pathophysiology: genetics, hormones, metabolism and beyond', *International Journal of Molecular Sciences*, Wawrzkiewicz-Jalowiecka et al., 2020

'Keeping egg cells fresh with epigenetics', babraham.ac.uk, 2018

'Mitochondrial dysfunction: an emerging link in the pathophysiology of polycystic ovarian syndrome', *Mitochondrion*, Shukla, 2020

'New findings about how a human egg matures may help prevent infertility and birth defects', ec.europa.eu, 2019

'Oxidative stress induces telomere shortening in human oocytes of advanced age donors', *Cells*, Kordowitzki et al., 2021

'PCOS and eating disorders in women', eatingdisorderhope.com, 2022

'Polycystic ovary syndrome: a brain disorder characterized by eating problems originating during puberty and adolescence', *International Journal of Molecular Sciences*, Steegers-Theunissen, 2020

'Polycystic ovary syndrome, insulin resistance and obesity: navigating the pathophysiologic labyrinth', *International Journal of Reproductive Medicine*, Rojas et al., 2014

'Risk of malignant ovarian cancer based on ultrasonography findings in a large unselected population', *JAMA Internal Medicine*, Smith-Bindman, 2018

TCP for Fallopian-tube conditions

'Abnormally increased DNA methylation in chorionic tissue might play an important role in development of ectopic pregnancy', *Reproductive Biology and Endocrinology*, Cai et al., 2021

'Attenuated tubal and endometrial urocortin 1 and corticotropin-releasing hormone receptor expression in ectopic pregnancy', *Reproductive Science*, Borges et al., 2011

'Corticotrophin releasing hormone and corticosterone impair development of preimplantation embryos by inducing oviductal cell apoptosis via activating Fas system', *Human Reproduction*, Tan et al., 2017

'Curvature in the reproductive tract alters sperm surface interactions', *Nature Communications*, Raveshi et al., 2021

'Egg transport and fertilization', GLOWM, Ghazal

'The tubal epigenome – an emerging target for ovarian cancer', *Pharmacology and Therapeutics*, Reavis et al., 2020

'Tubal transport of gametes and embryos: a review of physiology and pathophysiology', *Journal of Assisted Reproduction and Genetics*, Ezzati et al., 2014

TCP for conditions of the vagina

Girls and Sex, Peggy Orenstein, 2016

Vagina, Lynn Enright, 2019

Vagina, Naomi Wolf, 2012

'Adult-onset vulvodynia in relation to childhood violence victimization', *American Journal of Epidemiology*, Farlow et al., 2005

Bibliography

'Cancer and Mediterranean diet: a review', *Nutrients*, Mantella et al., 2019

'Characteristics of the vaginal microbiome in women with and without clinically confirmed vulvodynia', *American Journal of Obstetrics and Gynecology*, Bedford et al., 2020

'Immune mechanisms in vulvodynia: key role for mast cells and fibroblasts', *Frontiers in Cellular and Infection Microbiology*, Tonc et al., 2023

'Is chronic stress during childhood associated with adult-onset vulvodynia?', *Journal of Women's Health*, Khandker et al., 2014

'The preventative effect of dietary antioxidants on cervical cancer development', *Medicina*, Ono et al., 2020

'Psychological aspects associated with the acquisition and development of HPV infection and its repercussions on quality of life', *The Open Dermatology Journal*, Aragones et al., 2009

'Psychological aspects of cervical cancer', *Indian Journal of Psychological Medicine*, Kulhara et al., 1988

'Psychosocial stress and cervical neoplasia risk', *Psychosomatic Medicine*, Coker et al., 2003

'The vaginal microbiota, human papilloma virus and cervical dysplasia: a systematic review and network meta-analysis', *BJOG*, Norehang et al., 2020

Acknowledgements

I'm grateful to my patients over the years who have entrusted me with guiding them on their path to parenthood, for they have taught me so much, and some of their case studies are featured in this book, with their consent. I value and appreciate their honesty and willingness to share their stories and experiences, many of which touch on sensitive subjects, and their desire to help others facing similar situations in order to help alleviate their suffering. Their names and other features have been anonymized to respect their privacy, yet their stories remain as true as possible to the actual accounts; they know who they are, and I thank them wholeheartedly for allowing me to share their stories. A special mention goes to Kathryn and Dan, who not only shared their journey to parenthood on national TV, but also agreed to be a big part of this book. I'm humbled by the support they have shown me ever since I met them, and by their passion in wanting to help all those affected by similar challenges. And, of course, I'm forever grateful to my TV family on *This Morning*, who believed in and gave me the opportunity to bring The Conception Plan to all those who needed to hear and see it.

Thank you to my publisher, Penguin Life, which has supported me in all the challenges that come with writing a first book, and for believing in the bigger vision, even when at the start it all seemed difficult to piece together. Most of all, I thank them for trusting in me when I claimed that this genre needed something different, and that the face of medicine was changing to a more integrated path. I set out to write a book that I felt was missing, and I hope I've managed to do that. There are scores of people involved in publishing a book, but particular mention goes to Emily, Anya and Brigid for all their input in distilling the many complex and academic concepts into something accessible to all, and for helping to cut down what was originally a manuscript three times this size, even when it felt too painful to do so!

This book would not have been possible were it not for some

important people that I wish to mention, some of whose influence dates back several decades. I have to start with my teachers, in particular the ones who taught me English. When I first came to the UK aged eight, they helped me develop my love of the language and of the written word. I remember devouring copies of *Reader's Digest*, which my mum had on subscription back in the 1990s, and reading *Women's Bodies, Women's Wisdom* by Christiane Northrup, which my mum, herself a gynaecologist, bought when she saw Oprah recommend it on TV. Little did she know that the book would speak directly to me at the age of thirteen, and would go on to inspire what I came to do professionally.

Those small, seemingly inconsequential actions are what determined so much of my own fate, despite how mundane they seemed at the time. As my spiritual teacher says, magic is what happens in the everyday and what unfolds as we live our lives, doing the best we can, with every day that we get. That's what my parents unknowingly did all those years ago, and without their love and sacrifices I wouldn't be where I am today. I'm grateful to my whole family who realized my passion for writing from an early age and encouraged me on this path, keeping my very first stories I wrote as a child stacked somewhere in their treasure trove! They were the first people who taught me about the importance and meaning of family, along with my ancestors and relatives who all form part of my wider family, some of whom may not be here in physical form, but whose influence and inspiration are woven into the fabric of this book.

There are many friends and teachers who helped to support my vision of this book and who have come to feel a part of my extended family, encouraging me during the times when it felt too overwhelming and difficult, and being there for me as I underwent my own transformation during the writing. A special mention goes to Linda and Phil, Rena and Martin, Dominic, Lisa, Eliana, Bex and Matt, Bridget and John, Matt, Catie, Mauro and Katarina, Daisy, Emma, Safia, Maryanne, Ivka, Emma, Alice, Terezija and Max, Liz and Phoebe.

And then there are all the great teachers whose shoulders I stand upon, indebted to the legacies they have carved and their dedication and commitment to humanity, to become the thought leaders of today. They include: Christiane Northrup, Deepak Chopra, Bruce Lipton, Gabor Maté, Gregg Braden, Gabby Bernstein, Sister Joan Chittister and Zach Bush.

Finally, I have come to learn that as much as we value and appreciate the positive support of those who see the best in what we do, we must have equal gratitude for those who don't. I've had my fair share of those – people who undermined my views and ideas, as well as myself as a woman and a doctor. As difficult as it was to deal with this, I'm grateful to those people and the experience they gave me, as they helped me to come into the embodiment of the person I needed to be to write this book, helping to influence an emerging new paradigm of healthcare. Most of all, they meant that I had to trust my convictions and myself when I was made to feel like an outcast and understand that having faith in that which others can't necessarily see is a precious gift that may one day go on to help many others.

It's my sincerest desire that this book will help all those reading it and facing their own obstacles, to trust and to know that no matter how difficult the road gets, the wisdom and strength you build on the way are what will shape you and move the world around you. The act of wanting to become a parent is one of undeniable faith, courage and healing, and I hope this book becomes your treasured companion on this most sacred of paths.

Index

eggs and sperm 10, 15, 19–20, 22, 137, 254
  Juno–Izumo interaction 314
electromagnetics 128–9
embryo donation 255–6
embryos 40, 82, 86, 116, 123, 172, 207, 224–5
  chromosomal abnormalities 240, 257
  donation 255–6
  miscarriage 224–5, 226, 227
emotional cycle 268–70
Emotional Freedom Technique (EFT)
  72–3
emotional pain 33
emotional trauma 269–70
emotions 11–12, 29, 149, 223
  cellular level 33–4
  energy and 39–40
  feeling emotional 31–3
  healing 31, 32, 39–40
  infertility 53–4
  male fertility 211
  as messengers 54
  miscarriages 229–32
  negative 31–2
  predisposition to disease 32
  reproductive conditions 266–7
  stress management 116
  togetherness 189
  tools for processing
    breathwork 72
    therapies for trauma 72–3
  usefulness of 54
Endocrine Society 121–2
endocrine system 30–31, 267–8, 305
endometrial hyperplasia 79
endometriosis 32, 57, 79, 274–7
  case study 275–6
  changes in neurochemicals 63
  diagnoses 63, 64
  impact of 274
  inheritance 273
  osteopathy 45
  stress 63

  symptoms 274
  trauma 63–4
  vicious cycles of 276–7
endometrium 20
energetic body system 38–9
energetic healers 41
energies 37–8
  chakras 41–5
  emotions and 39–40
  energy–spirit–healing connection
    38–9
  meridian system 40–41
environmental oestrogens
  (xenoestrogens) 122
epi markers 21
epigenetic profile 9
epigenetics 17–24, 256
  changes 17–18
  constant communication 18–19
  difficulties conceiving 22–3
  impact on fertility 19–20
  implications for children 20–21
  legacy 21–2
epigenome 17, 18, 23, 27, 62, 135, 197, 224,
  273, 313–14
erectile dysfunction (ED) 89, 114, 122,
  209–11
exercise 4, 97–104, 214
  anti-ageing benefits 98
  assisted reproductive technology
    (ART) 103–4
  benefits of 97–9
  chronic endurance training 104
  enjoyment 99–101
  intensity 100–102
  male fertility 104
  during menstrual cycle 164–5, 283
  mitochondrial function 97–8
  moderation 100
  for ovarian conditions 305, 308–10
  recovery from miscarriage 233–4
  sex 183–4

PCOS (polycystic ovary syndrome) 15,
50, 55, 67, 79, 122, 227, 295
AGEs 82
causes of 297–8
contributory factors 296
diagnosis 296
eating disorders 302
emotional issues 32, 299–300
exercise 97, 99
psychological stress 297
reproductive conditions 262, 263,
264–5
TCP advice 307–10
pelvic inflammatory disease (PID) 51,
265, 313, 314, 318, 322
penis 132
Pennebaker, James W. 186–7
peptide YY 265
periods 3, 22, 27, 122, 159, 281
personal care 124–8
personality traits 55–6
pesticides 78, 79
PFAS (Perfluoroalkyl and
Polyfluoroalkyl Substances) 121
pheromones 137
phytochemicals 170–71
phytoestrogens 88
phytonutrients 80
Pilates 103
pill, the 27–8
pistachios 161
pituitary gland 206
placebo effect 28
plant-based milks 87
plant protein 87
plastic 126, 159
pleasurable sex 136–7
pleasure 178–81
PMS (premenstrual syndrome) 71–2
poleaxe hypothesis 138
polycystic ovaries 3, 31, 49, 296

polycystic ovary syndrome (PCOS)
see PCOS (polycystic ovary
syndrome)
polyps 279–80
pomegranates 183
pornography 210, 214
positive affirmations 34–5
post-natal depletion 69
potted plants 127
pre-eclampsia 77
pre-implantation genetic testing (PGT)
257
prebiotics 81, 169
preconception
alcohol 88–9
dealing with trauma 70
holistic approach 37
puberty 13–14
pregnancy
getting pregnant *see* conceiving
impact of trauma on babies 61
placenta 77, 122
preparing your body for 8–9
processed foods 77
smoking during 129–30, 205–6
stress during 61
pregnancy tests 3
premature ejaculation 99, 183, 210–11
premature menopause 246
prenatal period 61
prenatal supplements 146
probiotics 81–2, 87, 169, 173, 212, 266, 327
processed foods 77
meats 87, 308
vegetable oils 84–5
progesterone 31, 109, 110, 137, 178, 269,
286
prostatic fluid 206
protein 86–7, 169, 232
psychological resilience 62
psychotherapy 56